Are Your Teeth Killing You?

Are Your Teeth Killing You?

"Open Up"
This book could save your life.

Charles W. Martin, DDS

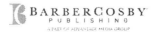
BARBERCOSBY
PUBLISHING
A PART OF ADVANTAGE MEDIA GROUP

Published by BarberCosby, Charleston, South Carolina.
Member of Advantage Media Group.

BARBERCOSBY is a registered trademark and the BarbyCosby colophon is a trademark of Advantage Media Group, Inc.
Printed in the United States of America.

ISBN: 978-1-59932-179-0
LCCN: 2010900779

This publication is designed to provide accurate and authoritative information in regard to the subject matter covered. It is sold with the understanding that the publisher is not engaged in rendering legal, accounting, or other professional services. If legal advice or other expert assistance is required, the services of a competent professional person should be sought.

Most Advantage Media Group titles are available at special quantity discounts for bulk purchases for sales promotions, premiums, fundraising, and educational use. Special versions or book excerpts can also be created to fit specific needs.
For more information, please write: Special Markets, Advantage Media Group, P.O. Box 272, Charleston, SC 29402 or call 1.866.775.1696.

Visit us online at **barbercosby**.com

Don't Lose Out,
Get More

Before you go any further... Please register your book now.

We have created an online companion to help you see, hear and feel the miracle of modern dentistry. The stone age of dentistry is long gone. You can have the smile you have always wanted in a comfortable and relaxed environment.

Register your Book at: http://ww.RegisterForMore.com to gain insider access to:

- Special offers
- Giveaways
- How to videos
- Insider information to upcoming events
- Patient success story videos and audios
- Actual patient before and afters
- Procedural videos
- Virtual tours
- and more...

Let us give you an online tour right now.

Register your Book at: http://www.RegisterForMore.com

If you have any questions, comments or concerns, please contact us at: info@RegisterForMore.com. We look forward to hearing from you.

Contact Us:

Richmond Smile Center
11201 Huguenot Rd
Richmond, VA 23235
Office: 804-320-6800
Fax: 804.320.1014
Email: info@RichmondSmileCenter.com

www.RichmondSmileCenter.com
www.MartinSmiles.com

Contents

Preface:

Common sense would tell you that what affects the mouth affects the rest of your body. In the case of oral health, common sense is too uncommon.

Strangely, the connections between the health or disease of the mouth and the rest of the body are NOT taught in medical schools, even today, in any depth. The separation of medical schools and dental schools, while advantageous for teaching, get's a big fat F when it comes to the public understanding and implication of diseases in the mouth and their connections to the rest of the body.

The appearance, smell, functional ability and biological indicators of health or disease in the mouth are often the first signs of problems in the body. Here are three quick examples:

- Chronic bad breath that won't go away can be a sign of gum disease and active infection with dozens of potentially harmful bacteria which are often found in the thickened and diseased blood vessels in and around the heart. If the bad breath that won't go away isn't caused by gum disease, then other body malfunctions may be detected. For example, your breath will smell different if you have uncontrolled diabetes.

- Upon examination, your dentist finds significant dental decay and general breakdown of your teeth. You were bewildered because you know that you eat well and take good general care of your teeth. Later, with more evaluation, you find that you were right all along. But you didn't know you had GERD, GastroEsophageal Reflux disease, with high acidity literally eating away your teeth. If you didn't know this you could have just given up and blamed it on bad genetics. Knowing the real reason, you can control your gastric reflux and keep your teeth and gums healthy.

- You notice your teeth are worn and they are getting worse. You often wake up with headaches and feel moody and grumpy during the day even though you get enough sleep. This could have easily gone undetected. An expert dentist would have questioned you about your sleep and breathing because when you experience excessive wear of your teeth, you often have sleep disordered breathing or Obstructive Sleep Apnea (OSA), which can be life threatening! Who knew of such things? Most people just don't make the connections.

There are dozens and dozens of examples like this throughout this book. Enjoy the reading, the explanations, and the new found knowledge. It just might mean the difference between healthy, happy living and a shortened, debilitated life. Isn't it better to know than to go blindly forward.

Happy reading,

Charles W. Martin, DDS

P.S. One comment made to me was, "Well, if my teeth can get me into so much trouble, wouldn't I just be better off without them?"

The instant and resounding answer is NO! Being without teeth worsens your ability to eat and over time causes facial disfigurement and a big fat drop in the quality of your life.

The mouth is where the health starts; where you smile, talk and eat. Its value is immense. Too often people neglect it. Then they discover what they lost and regret it. This book will help you to better understand your oral and total body health. What you don't know can hurt you, wouldn't you agree?

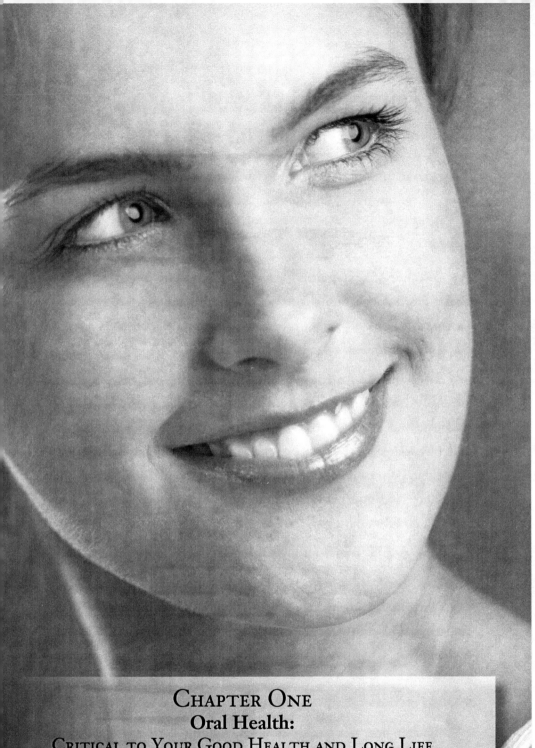

CHAPTER ONE
Oral Health:
CRITICAL TO YOUR GOOD HEALTH AND LONG LIFE

CHAPTER 1
Oral Health: Critical to Your Good Health and Long Life

A t one time in medical schools students were told to separate oral health from physical health. Most reacted with surprise. Who wouldn't think that what happens in the mouth affects physical health?

Because of that training, though, for quite a long time many health professionals didn't consider oral health and physical health to be linked. That's changed in recent years and now good oral health is being cited as important to physical health.

In 2006 the American Dental Association and the American Medical Association held a joint conference to discuss the benefits of medicine and dentistry working together. At the conference dentists and physicians focused on periodontal inflammation, diabetes and periodontal disease, oral infections and cardiovascular risk factors and pregnancy risks and periodontal disease. They also reviewed a new report linking smoking and root canals[1].

And recently oral health has also been linked to longevity[2].

But there's more news on the oral health front. I suspect this won't surprise any of my female readers but it may surprise a few male readers. Because men are more likely to ignore their oral health as well as their physical health you are also more likely to have dental problems associated with neglect, like tooth loss and gum disease[3]. And that can lead to a myriad of health problems and maybe even an early death.

Bottom line: oral health should be a serious concern for each and every one of us, male or female, no matter what age.

Good Dental Care Starts Early

Good dental care as a child can save you lots of time in the dental chair as an adult. Many adults who had poor dental care as children find that they spend much of their adult lives making up for that neglect. It's costly, it often takes a large investment of time and it's never as easy to repair damage as it is to prevent it.

If you're a baby boomer or older, you probably spent at least several of your early formative years without fluoridated water, especially if you lived in a rural area where most homes had well water. And you probably remember some dental techniques of that era that still make you flinch.

Fortunately dentistry has changed over the last few decades. And so has the quality of our oral health in the United States to some degree. But many people still suffer with dental problems that can easily be treated if caught early enough.

There are lots of reasons why we continue to have dental health problems in this country:

One issue is fluoride. Thirty eight percent of the U.S. population served by public water supplies don't have access to adequately fluoridated water4. And, if you drink bottled or filtered water you get very little fluoride.

Another issue is dental insurance. Many children who don't see a dentist regularly and who have dental problems that need treatment come from families that don't have dental insurance.

Then there's the issue of plain old fear of the dentist. I see it all the time. A patient may have had mostly good experiences with the dentist but one bad one leaves them scared of the next visit. Or a patient may have had lots of dental work as a child – in an era when pain was a mainstay of the dental experience – and as an adult decides that "I don't need to put myself through that." This is typically true of men who think they can stand a little pain. What most people don't realize is that pain in your mouth can have serious consequences.

Now if you look at TV at all, and most of us do, you'd think the only dental health issue in this country was finding the best whitening treatment to use to get a gleaming white smile!

Don't get me wrong. Gleaming white smiles are great. I try to make every patient that visits my office leave with teeth that look great. And I do a lot of cosmetic dentistry. But I also want my patients to have teeth that function the way they should and epitomize the ideal model of good oral health.

That requires regular check ups, treatment of minor gum disease before it becomes major, and good home dental care. Those are the basics. If you don't get a great set of teeth in the genetic gene pool, you may spend even more time in a dentist's office.

Regular Dental Care. Why Bother?

For some people the question is why bother? How about cutting your risk for diabetes, heart disease, kidney disease and cancer? Are those enough good reasons to start taking your dental care seriously? In 1998 the American Academy of Periodontology began working to educate the public on new research findings that linked infections in the mouth to problems in the rest of the body. Since then the research evidence continues to link gum disease to other diseases. While there's still a lot of research to be done, what has been completed suggests that gum disease contributes to the development of heart disease, increases your risk of stroke, increases a woman's risk of having a pre-term, low birth weight baby and poses a serious threat to people who have diabetes, respiratory diseases or osteoporosis.

Since a regular dental visit schedule will put you in the dentist's office more frequently than your annual physical puts you in your physician's office, we often see early signs of serious diseases. Believe me, if we do see early signs of serious disease, no matter what it is, we're going to pack you off to your physician right away. This means that the simple trip to the dentist that you were going to put off could save your life!

Equally important – it can help you save your teeth.   Dental problems start with bacteria – the bacteria that lurk in your mouth and cause tooth decay and gum disease if left to their own devices.   You mouth is like a condo complex for bacteria. They're in a snug, warm environment and the food you eat provides them food as well.   If you eat a lot of sugars then your mouth provides the bacteria that live in it with a series of endless desserts. The result? Tooth decay and gum disease that only gets worse if let go.

If you're thinking – I couldn't possibly have gum disease, I'd know it – think again.

In their early stages gum disease and infections rarely provide you with a clue that they are lurking in your mouth – there just aren't many symptoms. Yet it could be there. The National Institute for Health reports suggest that gum disease affects up to 80 percent of men and women in the United States.   It's one of the most prevalent microbial diseases known to man.   But it often goes undiagnosed .

Mild gum disease – called gingivitis – may leave you with red, swollen gums but it's not especially dangerous. At least not at first. But it can easily worsen into periodontitis and that is dangerous to the whole structure of your mouth.

That's bad enough. But remember this is an infection. And remember that stuff about how medical schools used to teach that the health body and the mouth are separate, not related? Well get a good periodontal infection going in your mouth and you'll quickly find out just how closely related your oral and physical health care.

Sure your system will fight a gum infection to try to keep it from spreading into other parts of the body. Frequently it succeeds, but when it doesn't the results can cause serious, long term damage or even kill you.

There are instances where gum disease bacteria have entered the bloodstream and moved to the heart, damaging heart valves. And we now believe that the resulting inflammation can release other infection-fighting compounds that can damage other tissues.

Your arteries are a common target. People with periodontal disease are twice as likely to die from heart attack and three times as likely to die from stroke.

I could go on and on about the dangers of not going to the dentist regularly and taking care of your oral health in between appointments. That's why I wrote this book. So let's move on to the next chapter where you'll learn more about periodontitis and the dangers of this nasty gum infection.

---

1 ADA, AMA collaborate on oral and systemic health media conference, http://www.ada.org/prof/resources/pubs/adanews/adanewsarticle.asp?articleid=1815, accessed 6/28/08

2 Why is Oral Health Important to Men?, Featured in Oral Health Resources, Men's Oral Health, Academy of General Dentistry, http://www.agd.org/support/articles/?ArtID=1266, accessed 6/26/08.

3 Ibid.

4 Dental Health: Flouride Treatment, Web MD, http://www.webmd.com/oral-health/guide/fluoride-treatment, accessed 6/28/08.

5 Mouth Body Connection, American Academy of Periodontology, www.perio.org/consumer/mbc.top2.htm, accessed 6/28/08.

What the Surgeon General reported

In 2000 the Surgeon General of the United States published the first Surgeon General's Report on Oral Health. The report went into great detail on the meaning of oral health and explained why oral health is so critical to our overall good health and well-being.

It was definitely a report whose time had come. The report talks about how during the previous 50 years great progress had been made in understanding and treating common oral health problems like tooth decay and gum disease. It discusses how those improvements made significant advances in the oral health of the general population. It also talks about how those improvements in oral health have changed attitudes – today most of us expect to keep our natural teeth for a lifetime. That wasn't the case 60, 70 or 100 years ago.

What pleased me most about this report, though, was the discussion of how oral health care had evolved from a focus on just the teeth and gums to the understanding that the mouth is the center of vital tissues and functions that affect our health and well being throughout our lives.

I've been saying that for years! It's your head! Why would anyone think what happens there is separate from the other parts of your body?

The major message of the report is that oral health is essential to the general health and well being of all United States residents. Even more important, it makes the point that good oral health can be achieved by all of us.

But, the report goes on to point out, not everyone living in the US has achieved an optimum level of oral health. Despite all the advances in dentistry and all the dental education that's taken place over the past 60 years or so many people still suffer needlessly from dental problems that affect their overall health, diminish their quality of life and, in some cases, may needlessly shorten their lives.

The Surgeon General's report describes the mouth as "a mirror of health or disease, as a sentinel or early warning system, as an accessible model for the study of other tissues and organs, and as a potential source of pathology affecting other systems and organs."[1] It goes on to say that a major theme of the report is that *oral health means much more than healthy teeth.*"[2]

What else does the Surgeon General list as necessary for oral health? It includes being free of:

- chronic oral-facial pain conditions,

- oral and throat cancers,

- oral soft tissue lesions,

- birth defects such as cleft lip and palate, and

- scores of other diseases and disorders that affect the oral, dental, and craniofacial tissues

Craniofacial tissues are the tissues that allow us to speak, chew, swallow and smile. They're also tissues the protect us against microbial infections and from many types of damage from the environment. And, as this report points out – many of the craniofacial tissues provide us with insight to organs and systems in less accessible parts of the body.

Examples include the salivary glands, which are a model of other exocrine glands. Jawbones and their joints function like other musculoskeletal parts. And the nervous system that affects facial pain is a model of nerves in other parts of the body.

The report also focuses on what can be detected in an oral exam – such as signs of nutritional deficiencies, diseases, infections, injuries, some cancers and some immune disorders. Examining the oral tissues, it says, provides a wealth of information about the rest of the body.

If you read the full report you'd find references to new research that associates chronic oral infections and heart disease, stroke, low birth weight babies and premature births. It also talks about the relationship between diabetes and gum disease, provides an assessment of these oral and systemic disease associations and an exploration of the mechanisms that may explain these connections.

This revised view of the importance of oral health in one's overall health is rewarding to those of us in the dental profession who've long seen the connections between what we saw going on in our patient's mouths and what they told us was going on in their bodies.

The only thing that surprises me is that it took nearly 50 years for the medical and dental professions to get to the conclusions drawn in the report. In 1948 the World Health Organization expanded the definition of health to mean "a complete state of physical, mental, and social well-being, and not just the absence of infirmity." Good oral health is part of that complete health definition. As we continue to research and learn more about the oral –systemic connection, I believe physicians and dentists will forge new relationships in their effort to care for the entire patient. Oral health is critical to your overall health. Don't ignore it.

---

1 US Department of Health and Human Services. Oral Health in America: A Report of the Surgeon General-- Executive Summary. Rockville, MD: US Department of Health and Human Services, National Institute of Dental and Craniofacial Research, National Institutes of Health, 2000.
2 Ibid.

Dan Kennedy
Arizona and Ohio

"Painless my behind."

How Dr. Charles Martin won over the "world's worst" dental patient

When Dan Kennedy called for a first appointment it was more like someone had slapped down the gauntlet and challenged me to defend my profession. Dan described himself as the "world's worst" dental patient and laid it all out for me. He was afraid of dentists, a demanding patient and assured me that he knew there was no such thing as "painless" dentistry. He challenged me to work on him and make it through the session with my professional confidence intact and my staff willing to continue working for me if he came back to the office. Here's Dan's story.

Dan Kennedy is an internationally known marking guru whose own Web page describes him as a "millionaire maker" for businesses of all kinds. Confident in all phases of business leadership, a well known public speaker and a direct mail and marketing guru who charges hundreds of dollars an hour for his consulting time, Dan was dentist phobic.

Before I ever met him, he told me he'd tried seven different dentists all over the United States who focused on patients who were afraid of the dentist – you've seen the dental ads that read "we cater to cowards." By the time I saw Dan, he needed gum surgery, bone grafts, root canals and bridge work. This was a challenging, multi-session effort we were embarking on.

Frankly he was scared. I think he'll admit that. The dentistry he'd tried had been billed as painless and it wasn't And Dan, who describes himself as "difficult" and as "a critical person" and adds "I complain constantly," told me he'd been banned from ever returning to these dentist's offices after just one visit each.

Well I make that promise of painless dentistry, too, and I mean it. And Dan was quick to tell me that I didn't quite live up to that promise. But he did admit that it was close to painless. Dan and I worked together over seven sessions to get his mouth back in shape. It was demanding, detailed dentistry with lots of invasive procedures that are never pleasant for any patient. Yet Dan admitted that while it wasn't painless, in the first five of the seven sessions he spent with me, he only needed one pain pill.

That was rewarding to hear as Dan had told me about his previous experience trying to get his dental problems corrected. He ended up swollen, bleeding for hours and in pain all night. It was three days before he could eat and his pain pill count was "handfuls." I'm truly proud of being able to turn that around for him 180 degrees.

When you work with someone like Dan you need to help him past his fear and tension. With him we used headphones with music, added a massage pad to the dental chair and included breaks whenever he needed them.

Other patients who need less work than Dan really do have painless sessions. Admittedly, no dentist can avoid occasionally causing a patient pain. But if you grew up in the '50s and '60s and remember dentistry as it was back then, rest assured that you

ARE YOUR TEETH KILLING YOU

should never have to experience the dental discomfort you had as a child.

For people like Dan who are diabetic, ignoring your dental care for many years carries a lot of danger – and the threat of premature death from diabetes-related conditions that are worsened by ignoring gum and other periodontal problems. So it's important to use as much new technology as possible to limit the possible amount of pain that someone like Dan experiences.

Dan's experience is what our entire office team seeks to accomplish in treating all patients. Like many of my patients, he'd had dental experiences that were all too common – driving him away from dentists for years and creating a situation in his mouth that took extensive work to correct. Experiences like Dan's have been a major inspiration in the creation of a nationwide organization of elite professionals who have in-depth knowledge about meeting unique oral and physical health needs of many patients who have found traditional treatment frustrating and challenging.

We practice complete transparency, explaining every procedure so you understand both the need for it and how it's done. We also focus on your comfort and, while we can't guarantee all of our procedures will be 100 percent pain-free, we do promise we'll make every effort to treat tender gum tissues with the utmost care as we work to return your oral health to the same robust status you enjoyed before periodontitis.

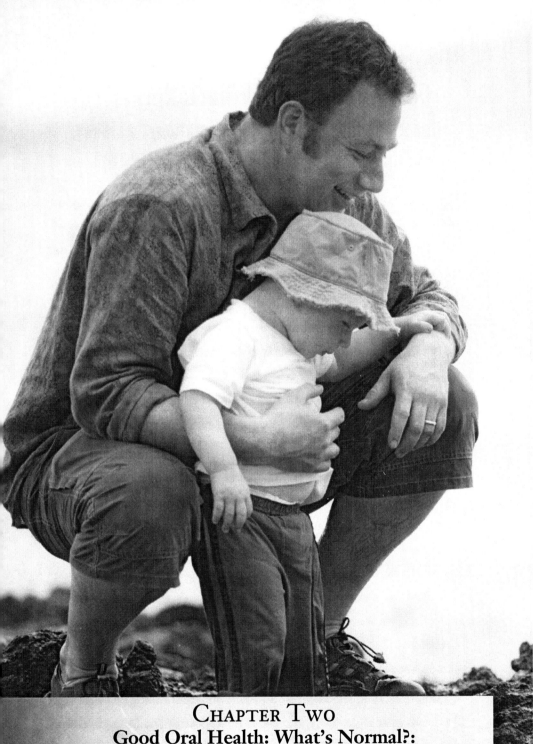

CHAPTER TWO
Good Oral Health: What's Normal?:
UNDERSTANDING SYSTEMIC INFLAMMATION, ITS LINKS
TO GUM DISEASE, AND ITS ROLE IN YOUR HEALTH

CHAPTER 2
Good Oral Health: What's Normal?
Understanding Systemic Inflammation, Its Links to Gum Disease, and Its Role in Your Health

B efore we get any further, let's clarify one very basic fact about normal oral health. This is a fact that holds true regardless of your health status, whether you're dealing with chronic disease or otherwise as healthy as a horse.

I can't begin to count the number of times a patient has come in for a regular checkup thinking that all is well when, in reality, they already have a periodontal disease. When I ask them whether they've noticed any symptoms they frequently say, "Well, there was a little blood a couple of times when I flossed and brushed, but it was only a trace and it doesn't happen all the time so I just figured that's normal."

There's nothing normal about blood in your mouth. For some reason, we're able to persuade ourselves that a trace of blood now and then while brushing or flossing doesn't indicate there's something wrong. That's one of the most common dental health myths out there today, and for the life of me I can't figure out where it comes from. After all, if we combed our hair and our scalp started to bleed even just a little bit most of us would wonder what's going on up there. Chances are we would at least call our doctor to see if we should get it checked out. And, of course, your doctor is going to want to take a look because that's not normal.

If you see even the slightest bit of blood after flossing or brushing, call your dentist right away and make an appointment for a checkup. This is particularly important if you have diabetes or have prediabetes.

Blood, no matter how small the quantity, is a sure sign that you have a gum problem that your dentist needs to examine. Right now!

Don't wait, because even if you don't see blood again for weeks that doesn't mean the problem has taken care of itself. It hasn't. Chances are it's getting worse and will eventually develop into a serious periodontal disease that will be more difficult to treat, more expensive to treat and uncomfortable to live with.

Prevention is much easier, and it's much better for your health.

Okay, I'm off my soapbox. Let's get into the details of how gum disease works, which sets the stage for a complete understanding of how periodontitis and other diseases together are a serious potential threat to your health.

Understanding What's In Your Mouth – And What's Going On In There

When we look in our mouth most of us see the usual assortment of equipment – teeth, gums and tongue. While the tongue can harbor bacteria that can be a problem, what we're mostly concerned with here are the teeth and gums. Actually, there's a lot more equipment that you can't see, yet it's vital to keep it all in proper working order to preserve good oral health.

Don't worry – I'm not going to try to make you sit through a n course in Dentistry 101. We're just going to cover the highlights in broad strokes so you have an understanding of how all this works.

The **cementum** is the outer layer on the roots of your teeth. It's a fairly thin layer, a sort of dull pale yellow, and it has two main jobs – to

Cementum

protect the root of the tooth, and to provide a solid surface to attach to the tissue that holds your tooth in place.

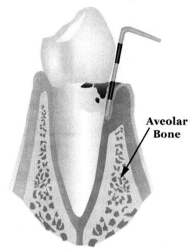

Aveolar / Bone

The **alveolar bone** is the socket that your tooth sits in. It's actually two bones — one is the socket itself and the other is a structural support, sort of like the joists that sit on beams to provide support for the floor in your house. This structure provides a firm anchor point for your tooth.

Periodontal ligaments are connective tissues that do just that — they connect the cementum and the gum to the alveolar bone.

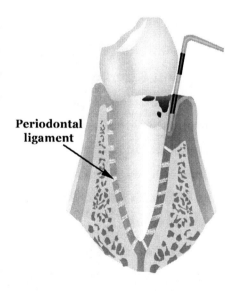

Periodontal ligament

Working together, this team of components keep your teeth stable so they can do all the crushing, tearing and grinding that we give little conscious thought to as we enjoy every meal.

We could keep on going and cover some of the finer details, but *these are the basics*.

The whole structure described here is covered by the gum. Well, it's pretty well covered in healthy teeth. But the trouble begins when plaque starts to accumulate at the gum line. As the plaque keeps building up, some of the bacteria that make up the plaque can work their way under the gum line. That's a nice, cozy location where bacteria can thrive because it's hard for you to reach them with floss or your toothbrush.

In fact, it's so cozy that the term "hog heaven" might well have been coined to describe what a great life the bacteria are having down under the gum line. Think of it as a sort of Utopian condominium complex for bacteria. It's snug, warm, moist, there's plenty of room and initially there are very few problems in the neighborhood. They even have a bountiful supply of food from actual food particles that are trapped in the plaque.

At any one time your gums and your teeth are hosting hundreds of different bacteria. Happy and comfortable, these bacteria carry on their busy lives and multiply profusely. They don't let up at any time – they're carrying out their little party in your mouth 24/7. As a byproduct of their lifestyle, they produce toxins. You might think of these toxins much like the trash we throw into the wastebasket under the sink and empty on a regular basis so odors don't develop. The problem under the gum line is there's no way to take out the trash.

Inflammation Is the Key

As these bacteria continue to build and secrete toxins, the toxins accumulate and – because they aren't getting cleaned out – begin to irritate the neighboring gum tissue.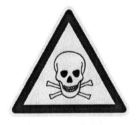

Sensing the irritation, the body responds with an automatic system that's a defense mechanism against inflammation. This is referred to as the body's inflammation response, a complex set of events that send several different types of cells to the site. These cells have specific jobs that are designed to remove whatever is causing the irritation and help the tissue that's been injured to start to heal.

The longer the inflammation continues, the more the body's inflammation response system sends more cells and different types of cells into the battle. (And remember, any one of these bacteria at any time can lead to inflammation and infection so your mouth may be hosting a battle that beats any legendary battle played out in the movies or on TV.) The harder the fighting gets, the more the surrounding tissue gets injured.

It's bad enough to have this going on in your mouth all by itself. But if you are fighting a chronic disease like diabetes it's even worse because of the dangers bacterial infections pose for many chronic diseases. In the specific case of people who have diabetes, these little partiers are thriving on the sugar you have trouble regulating. They're not just having a party in your mouth, they're enjoying unlimited servings of multiple desserts.

How can you know if this is going on in your mouth? Well you may feel some soreness, you might see the area get red and you could experience some swelling. In a pitched battle, when the inflammatory response cells mount a major counterattack against the bacteria, you may develop an infection as the body's cells try to surround, contain and ultimately destroy the enemy.

Although this sounds like one single process, there are many things going on at the same time while the body tries to respond to fight off the bacteria and reduce the inflammation. You may hear your dentist talk about a cascade of events that trigger a series of health effects throughout your body.

It starts, of course, with the local situation in your mouth, where the bacteria and its toxins are attacking your periodontal structures. Remember the gum, the cementum, the alveolar bone and the periodontal ligaments? As the bacteria continue to expand their foothold under the gum line, they cause more and more damage to your gum, which can begin to pull away from your tooth. As the gum recedes and

forms open pockets around your teeth, the bacteria have more room to multiply. They also have a clearer path to the other parts of the interlocking system that protect and anchor your teeth. The cementum fails, there's a loss of bone in the socket that cradles the tooth, and the ligaments that connect these parts together are loosened or pulled away. The end result is that your gums are

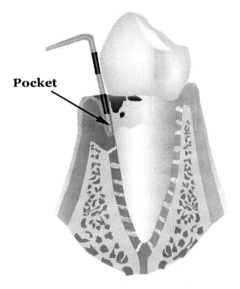

Pocket

inflamed and sore, and your teeth are no longer stable. The risk of permanent tooth loss may now be very real unless you go to your dentist for treatment. You may even run the risk of serious infection below the gum, as well as the potential for the actual death of gum, bone and connective tissues.

For more about periodontal diseases see "What Is Periodontitis?"

Systemic Inflammation Means Serious Health Risks

The problem with the kind of inflammation that is triggered by gum disease is that it doesn't stay in the mouth. Remember the hundreds of oral bacteria we just mentioned? A number of them are bad actors, pathogens that can cause infection, inflammation and disease.

Some of them can get into your bloodstream and spread far and wide throughout your body.

The result is something called chronic systemic inflammation. It's an emerging field in many healthcare specialties. Given all the research that's going on today – there are literally hundreds of articles in professional journals about scientific research into this area – I'm positive you're going to hear more and more about it in the popular media.

This inflammation reminds me of a spy thriller mystery on the order of a Tom Clancy novel, or even an Ian Fleming book featuring James Bond. There's a hidden enemy lurking undercover, undetected yet doing its dirty work throughout your body, all the while staying under the radar even as its damage continues to compound. Think of the body's inflammation response as the physiological stand-in for Sean Connery, dashing to the rescue just when it seems that the nefarious scheme for total body domination is building to a climactic fevered pitch.

The secret weapons that stop this dastardly plot in its tracks are elements of the body's immune system, battling infections with wave upon wave of different types of cells. Unfortunately, like a Hollywood scriptwriter who can't resist overly melodramatic lines for leading characters, the body's responses can shift into overdrive, resulting in too much of a good thing. That, in turn, can damage various organs and systems, leading to serious health complications and potentially catastrophic health events.

As this story unfolds throughout the book – minus the literary metaphors – it will become increasingly clear that inflammation and infection that has its roots in gum disease can wreak havoc at virtually any location throughout the body. This cascade of inflammation and the body's reactions contribute to some diseases and conditions, and actually cause others.

The really insidious part of the problem is that it is so far beneath the surface, nearly invisible to even the trained professional, rarely rising to the level of a readily diagnosed symptom, that it's often overlooked. Yet, when it's treated, brewing health problems can be prevented and existing conditions may be resolved.

As a result of reading this book and its detailed discussion of the links between oral health, inflammation, the immune response and many health risks, you'll be better prepared to talk with your health care professionals about considering the role these factors may play in your personal well-being.

Are You At Risk Of Periodontal Disease? Take This Risk Test And Find Out!

The American Academy of Periodontology, a national association of gum disease specialists, has a brief test that lets you know how much risk you run of having periodontal disease.

You'll have the answer after just 12 quick questions.

The test is available on the Web at:

http://service.previser.com/aap/default.aspx.

What Is Periodontitis?

Put in its most simple terms, periodontitis is gum disease. The literal meaning of the word 'periodontal' is straightforward – 'peri' means 'around', and 'dont' means 'tooth'. So, periodontal refers to the parts of your mouth that surround your tooth.

The word 'periodontitis' refers to the diseases that affect these parts of your mouth. These are generally bacterial infections that attack the gums and other oral components.

While periodontitis is generally used to refer to gum disease, there are other parts of your mouth that are considered part of your periodontal structures. These include the bone that supports your teeth and the tissues that connect your teeth to the bone.

Periodontists are dentists who specialize in preventing and treating these infections.

Periodontal diseases take several forms, including these common types.

- **Gingivitis** is a mild form of gum disease. You may hear dental health professionals refer to the 'gingiva'. That's the clinical term for your gums. Gingivitis often develops when plaque builds up on your teeth at the gumline and irritates the gum. The irritation makes it easier for bacteria to infect gum tissue. The infection inflames the gum, which can then become red, swell up around your teeth, and bleed easily. Gingivitis is easily treated. If you let gingivitis go untreated, it can turn into periodontitis.

- **Aggressive periodontitis** happens in otherwise healthy people who have a bacterial infection in their gums that continues to worsen until it destroys the supporting bone and your teeth begin to loosen.

- **Chronic periodontitis** is more severe. Bone loss and loosening gets worse, the gums pull away from your teeth and pockets can form around your teeth where the gum used to be. This traps even more plaque and bacteria, which just adds more fuel to the fire.

- **Necrotizing periodontitis** is as bad as it sounds. This is a condition in which parts of your gum, bone and connective tissues can actually die.

The American Academy of Periodontology, a national association of gum disease specialists, has a brief test that lets you know how much risk you run of having periodontal disease. The test is available on the Web at http://service.previser.com/aap/default.aspx.

Bacteria: The good, the bad and the ugly

They're in your mouth!

Bacteria in your mouth are a fact of life. They cause tooth decay and they cause gum disease, both of which are controllable with regular dental check ups. Yeah, I know you've heard that all your life, but hear me out.

What I see every day are people who don't get regular dental check ups. And eventually the bacteria get out of control, damaging teeth and gums. Until it gets really serious lots of people never know they have these types of infections. There are few symptoms and often little pain.

It's a routine: brush, floss and see your dentist regularly to make sure any developing problems are caught quickly and treated.

But is that what's really happening? Lots of people are more concerned with a brilliant smile – not surprising given the push for teeth-whitening systems we've seen in recent years – than they are with making sure they get to the dentist regularly. And they're focused on that, often using in-home treatments while avoiding the routine cleaning and polishing.

Lots has improved in oral health in the United States in recent decades with treatments like dental sealants for kids and reports about lower rates of tooth decay in permanent teeth in just the last few years.

But a report from the Centers for Disease Control and Prevention recently confirmed that one in three Americans over 30 has advanced gum disease or periodontitis, nine of ten Americans have some tooth decay and three of 10 adults over 65 have no teeth at all.

Diabetes is just one of many diseases that are sometimes first diagnosed in the dentist's office. Others include Crohn's disease, skin diseases, autoimmune diseases and cancer. And untreated dental woes can sap your energy. A mouth infection demands a constant fight response from the body, a sure way to wear you out.

Some 35 percent of all Americans over age two haven't been to a dentist in over a year. We dentists sometimes wonder if people forget that their head is attached to the rest of their body. Yet healthy teeth and gums are one of the greatest self-esteem boosters in the world. It's your smile, take care of it!

Testimonial - In Their Own Words - Childhood Dental Problems

When childhood dental problems dog you into adulthood.

It's not unusual to have a patient whose childhood dental problems plague him or her into adulthood. Maybe it's the fear induced by some of the less than gentle dental procedures of the early and mid-twentieth century, maybe it's poor prenatal care a patient's mother received, maybe it's someone who came from a family that found it difficult to afford dental care.

Whatever reason, many patients spend their adult years making up for lost time. Here's what Virginia Miller to say about how quality dental care as an adult has helped her.

"When I was born the good teeth gene was missing from my gene pool. I grew up during hard times when dental hygiene was not a priority. Surviving was the most important thing. With my uneven, crooked teeth my smile was always covered with my hand. One of the first things I did when I went to work was to have my front teeth capped. Now I could smile.

"Over the years I spent a lot of time in the dentist chair. My dread of having to have dentures was a constant nightmare for me. Then it happened! My teeth started breaking off. Just broke right off when I was chewing something. The first one I put into a small cup in the medicine cabinet and the next one and the next. Why I saved them I do not know. Perhaps it was my way of thinking they were not really gone. My dentist at that time did not know what to do. I went to different dentists, one for this problem, one for another problem. I had some teeth extracted.

Then I learned I had gum disease. So I said to myself, 'This is serious. Your entire health could be in jeopardy.'

"I knew I needed to take serious action. I still had the teeth in my medicine cabinet, the teeth I was losing were getting closer to the front of my mouth and my smile was in danger as was my health.

"I considered implants. When I went to see Dr. Martin, whose work with implants I'd read about, I was very impressed – especially since I could get all the work done in his office. He advertised friendly, gentle dentistry and he came through on that promise.

"Even so, I was nervous and apprehensive. My history with other dentists made me cautious, but Dr. Martin lived up to his advertising. Not only was he gentle, the procedures were essentially painless.

"Dentistry has made amazing progress in the last few years and it's great to have a dentist who keeps up to date. I now have teeth to chew with and a smile I'm proud to display."

Virginia, like many people who came up during hard times, has committed to improving her health and her smile with reconstructive dentistry that fixes the problems of the past so that our patients can enjoy a healthy, smiling future.

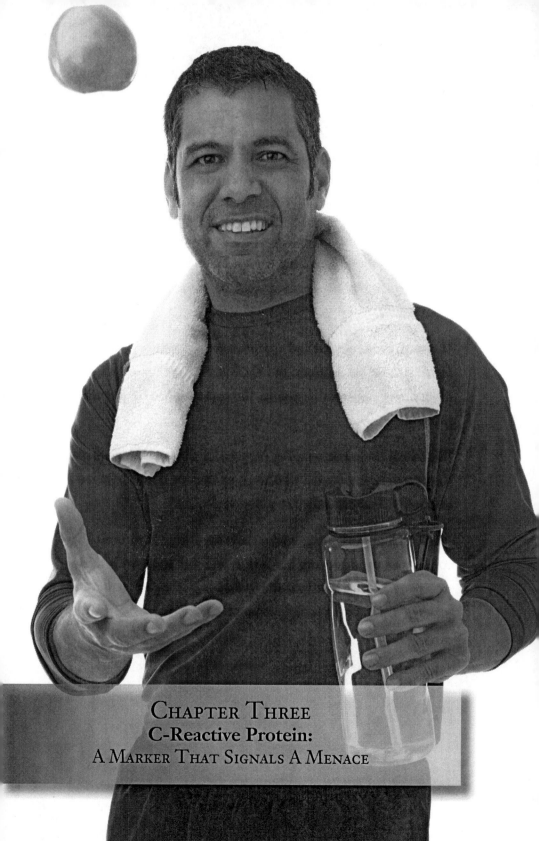

CHAPTER THREE
C-Reactive Protein:
A MARKER THAT SIGNALS A MENACE

CHAPTER 3
C-Reactive Protein: A Marker That Signals a Menace

C-reactive Protein (CRP) is a protein that is present in your blood plasma when your body senses inflammation. It's used by doctors as an inflammation marker, a way to tell that even though you may not know it yet and it may not be visible, your body is fighting inflammation somewhere.

CRP is produced by the liver, but only under certain circumstances. In normal, healthy people CRP may not even show up in a blood test. But when the body starts fighting inflammation, it starts sending a variety of cytokines that carry different messages to cells in many locations. These messenger cells are sort of like the body's Paul Revere, riding from place to place to wake up the militia and spring them into action. Some of the messengers will alert other cells and tell them that there's an emergency somewhere in the body and they need to go to work doing whatever their part is in the body's myriad ways of responding to a threat. Other messengers tell the cells how to interact with another group of cells to fight the inflammation, in effect giving the cells marching orders, sending them to the front, and telling them when and where to attack.

One of these messengers heads directly to your liver, sounding the alarm about the inflammation and telling it to crank up its production line because the body needs C-reactive protein for some specific purpose. Interestingly enough, we don't know all the details yet about exactly what that purpose is. Right now, what we do know is that CRP is pumped into the blood when the body experiences inflammation. Whether CRP has a more active role in fighting inflammation is something that researchers are still trying to discover. They're also taking a long, hard look at whether CRP is something of a villain. It may, in fact, turn out be a bad guy that contributes to some major health problems.

So, what causes the inflammation that rings all these alarm bells throughout the body? Well, gum disease, for one. The bacteria that cause gingivitis and periodontitis flip every switch that the body has built into its inflammatory response mechanisms and turn on all its natural defenses. We talked earlier in some detail about how that works, so there's no need to go through it again.

This inflammation alone can worsen your gum disease. As the periodontitis develops into progressively more serious stages, it can pile its inflammation on top of the atherogenesis. This whole process can compound the cycle even further, as well as worsen a number of serious health conditions.

Atherogenesis is the process of forming plaques on the inner lining of the arteries. As the plaques pile up and spread across the arterial walls, they irritate the lining and cause inflammation.1 Even though it's not caused by bacteria or other organisms, inflammation is inflammation. Without fail and without regard to the source, it triggers the body's inflammatory response, and the whole cascade of adverse health events that go along with it.

And, as if this wasn't enough, extensive research into CRP has shown that it's associated with a wide variety of health risks and events. These include high cholesterol, hardening of the arteries, heart disease, even mental health problems. Note that I said it's associated with these things, not necessarily that it causes them. Research hasn't determined that yet.

CRP and Heart Disease: It's a Predictor. Is It Also a Cause?

It's an established fact that high CRP levels can consistently predict heart attack and stroke, as well as death from cardiovascular disease. In fact, the higher your CRP level is, the less likely you are to survive one of these catastrophic events.[2]

If your CRP level climbs into the upper third of the measurement category, your risk of having a heart attack is two times that of people whose CRP level is in the lower third.[3] The research showed that this was true for men, women, and the elderly.

For those who have already had a balloon angioplasty, which is a procedure to open up a blocked artery and restore better blood flow, CRP levels can be used to predict whether the artery will close up again.[4]

These are not trivial risks. Elevated CRP levels carry an increased risk of coronary heart disease for the next 10 years. This is associated with just the mere presence of CRP, regardless of whether you have any of what we typically think of as cardiac risk factors. Just one single CRP measurement can provide additional diagnostic information beyond conventional risk assessments for heart disease.[5]

One study showed that CRP is at least as effective as cholesterol levels as a predictor of cardiovascular risk.[6] Other researchers even found CRP to be better than cholesterol as a predictor of heart disease.[7]

A lot of recent research suggests that CRP at least contributes to the buildup of plaque that causes blood clots in arteries. Now, researchers have conclusively linked CRP to the formation of blood clots.[8] CRP appears to affect endothelial cells, which are the flat cells that form the lining of arteries. CRP causes these cells to release an enzyme that is a marker for blood clot development. It also keeps other compounds from breaking down the clot. This has significant implications for both blood clots and all of the major health problems that clots can cause. [9] Blood clots, of course, cause everything from strokes to pulmonary embolisms to heart attacks – all of which can easily be fatal.

Some research also indicates that CRP may provide a novel method for detecting people who are at high risk of plaque rupture.[10] This is important because if we can lower the risk of arterial plaques breaking up and sending a clot, or even a shower of clots, into the bloodstream where they can block blood flow to the heart, lungs or brain we can then reduce the likelihood of heart attack or stroke.

So, in addition to being a marker for inflammation, is CRP a cause of health problems? The research isn't rock-solid on this yet. One of the latest research studies indicates that CRP is not the cause of chronic heart disease, but other researchers don't believe it's definitively ruled out as a cause.[11] What we are confident of is that CRP is a marker of major health risks. It alerts your physician to the presence of inflammation and inflammation, experts believe, is likely to be the cause of chronic heart disease. Personally, I believe that future research will link CRP to a variety of chronic health problems. Stay tuned as the research continues!

All of this also tends to confirm previous research that suggested that low-grade inflammation is involved in atherosclerosis, the progressive thickening and hardening of the walls of medium and large arteries.[12] In fact, we already know that CRP is related to arterial stiffness in otherwise healthy people as well as those who have system-wide inflammation in their blood vessels.[13] Studies also show that arterial stiffness increases in people who have a chronic system-wide inflammation.[14] I believe we'll find the same link there between inflammation-causing diseases such as diabetes and gum disease, and CRP.

Researchers have discovered that CRP increases the size of health disasters called infarcts. These are areas of tissues that die because they are starved of oxygen due to blockages in your arteries. When these occur in the heart muscle, you have a myocardial infarction, or heart attack. In the brain, it's a cerebral infarct, or stroke. Reducing or eliminating CRP is a promising indication that the probable underlying cause – inflammation – is also reduced, meaning less risk to your heart and brain from blood vessel blockages.[15]

One study showed that intensive treatment with statin drugs, such as Lipitor, produced greater reductions in both LDL cholesterol and CRP than the moderate statin treatment that is more typically prescribed. The scientists noted that this suggests a relationship between these two markers and the progression of coronary artery disease.[16]

CRP levels are also associated with future development of hypertension, or high blood pressure, which is one of the risk factors for several chronic diseases. This suggests that hypertension is in part an inflammatory disorder.[17] CRP and blood pressure have both been identified as independent indicators of cardiovascular risk. Now, researchers have found that their predictive value is additive. That means if you have both high blood pressure and a measurable level of CRP, your risk of heart attack is much higher than if you had just one of those indicators. The researchers who discovered this also concluded that increasing levels of blood pressure may kick the body's inflammatory response system into high gear.[18]

As it turns out, after surveying all the current research and looking at new areas that are being explored, CRP is being linked to a broad array of health issues. For example, CRP can even be used to identify a person's risk of developing colon cancer.[19] Other researchers have found that higher levels of cynical distrust and chronic stress were associated with higher levels of CRP.[20] There's no doubt that the list will increase as science improves our understanding of all that CRP does in the body.

The Good News – Periodontal Treatment Reduces CRP

Let's bring this all back to where we started – gum disease, inflammation and CRP. It's clear that these are all intertwined in a cascade of increasing health risks. The question is what to do about it.

Fortunately, we also have research showing that when you treat gum disease, CRP levels go down and, as a result, may decrease the risk of heart attack or stroke.[21] It's a good thing, because there is a direct link between periodontal disease and higher system-wide levels of CRP.[22] It's also been shown that heart attack survivors who suffer advanced gum disease show significantly higher levels of CRP.[23]

Specific methods of treating periodontal disease – using scaling and root planing combined with a topical antibiotic gel – are proven to significantly lower the levels of CRP associated with a heightened risk of heart disease.[24] These techniques may sound intimidating but they are less painful than what will surely develop into ever more severe gum disease and all the problems related to inflammation if left untreated. We'll go into detail about these procedures later. For now, it's important to know that when you treat the gum disease you also reduce all the associated risks from system-wide inflammation, CRP, and the compounding effects of all of these upon your overall health.

A relatively new tool in the dentist's CRP-fighting arsenal is antioxidant nutrients. Oxidative stress is caused when the body produces more free radicals than it can normally handle. Free radicals are oxygen-related byproducts of normal metabolism. Obviously, we need oxygen to survive, literally from breath to breath. But these cells are created as the body uses oxygen and sugar to produce the energy it needs simply to keep going. These free radicals, unchecked, damage surrounding molecules. The body usually has a supply of antioxidants that it uses to control the harm done by free radicals and to repair any damage. So, when the supply of antioxidants gets low the damage done by free radicals mounts up, causing inflammation. As the inflammation grows, CRP is released into the bloodstream, and you already know the rest of that story.

Recent research has demonstrated that antioxidant nutrients can keep the free radicals in check and reduce the inflammation. That, in turn, reduces the level of CRP in your blood. This is especially important because the cascade of effects caused by oxidative stress can be triggered by many risk factors for cardiovascular disease. It may, in fact, be the common thread that ties them all together.[25]

Antioxidants, generally taken in the form of supplements, are found in a wide variety of naturally healthy foods including a lot of fruits and vegetables. One of the most commonly used antioxidants is found in grape seed extracts.

There has been a lot of controversy over antioxidants, most of it due to the monumental struggle between mainstream pharmaceutical companies, nutraceutical manufacturers and the U.S. Food and Drug Administration. The FDA is correctly concerned about making sure that nutraceutical claims can be backed up, but the more research that is done the more the findings are confirming that these supplements can, indeed, play a major role in maintaining the body's normal structure and function. It's clear to me that in the not too distant future we'll see a lot more collaboration, as the pharmaceutical industry embraces nutraceuticals and forms entire new product lines featuring them. I can assure you that if your dentist combines your periodontal therapy with nutraceuticals that contain antioxidants, you can be sure that they have studied the supplement thoroughly and believe it will play an important part in reducing CRP levels and restoring your health.

Should You Have a CRP Test?

After reading all this detailed information about gum disease, inflammation, and CRP you may wonder how you can use this knowledge to improve your health. The question that seems logical is, "Should I have my CRP level checked?"

The American Heart Association and the U.S. Centers for Disease Control and Prevention have jointly studied the issue of CRP testing. Soon after the test became widely available, many active health consumers who had heard about it flocked to their physicians. In the absence of any formal guidance on the test, doctors ordered them for tens of thousands of their patients.

Many of these patients – probably most, in fact – were not experiencing any particular cardiovascular-related risks. For those patients, the AHA and CDC said, there is really no need to test CRP levels.

But the experts said that, for patients in the moderate risk category and above, CRP levels can provide medical professionals a better diagnostic view of their condition and may lead to more intensive treatment.[26]

The key, then, is to know your risk category for cardiovascular disease. The best way to determine that is to talk with a health care professional, such as your physician. Dentists who are certified through certain types of specially focused clinical training are also able to provide guidance about this risk and whether you should have a

CRP blood test done. And, if it appears that you are in the moderate risk group or higher, they can also have the test performed and interpret the results.

Here's what to look for if you and your doctor – whether it's your physician or your dentist – decide that you should have your CRP level tested. The test itself is called the highly sensitive C-reactive protein test, hs-CRP for short. The results are expressed in terms of milligrams of CRP per liter, which is written as mg/L.

Results indicate a low risk if the level of CRP is less than 1 mg/L. A level of 1 – 3 mg/L indicates an average risk. Above 3 mg/L is considered high risk. If you're in the high-risk group, you have about twice the risk of cardiovascular disease as those in the low-risk group.

Getting this kind of test can be scary. While you're waiting for your results, it's not uncommon to imagine the worst. My best advice is to just relax until you actually see the results. After all, if you're in the low or average-risk groups, there's probably nothing to worry about. Your doctor may want to keep an eye on the levels and do additional testing to make sure that it's not rising.

Even if you're in the high-risk group, there's still good news – and that is now you and your doctor know exactly what's going on in your body. That's the first crucial step to treating the inflammation so you can avoid the potential health risks that CRP signals.

I can also share with you my experience in treating patients who have gum disease. We take an initial CRP level before beginning treatment and another level at the end of the process. That gives us a benchmark of where we started so we can compare the results, a straightforward before and after measurement. We always use the hs-CRP test, which is highly sensitive and provides the most accurate results. It's typical to see someone who has periodontal therapy watch their CRP level take a dive – generally down to 3 or less!

I hope you find a substantial amount of comfort in the knowledge that together, you and your dentist can regain control over your gum disease and improve your health so you can enjoy a normal lifestyle for years to come.

Testimonial - Hilda Wilson

"Chewing is the best reward."

Chewing apples, carrots and celery again has been a great reward for Hilda Wilson after her dental treatment. Hilda came to our practice a few years ago and here is her story.

"At age 70, my dental concerns were more about chewing than about smiling. With improper care as a youngster, I lost a number of teeth interfering with my chewing surfaces. As the last chewing surface went, I was forced to make some replacement choices.

"After some discussions with other dentists, I resorted to the telephone directory. 'Friendly, Gentle Dentistry' appealed to me. At that point it was Dr. Charles Martin to the rescue.

"We discussed an overall dental plan. My requirement for satisfaction was that I not have any removable dental parts. Dr. Martin obliged. It involved five implants and at least six crowns – extensive and expensive work. I needed confidence and money! Dr. Martin's staff, who I experienced to be not only friendly to me, but also pleasant to each other (a comforting situation to a new patient), helped build my confidence.

"At first the whole procedure seemed too expensive. Eventually after researching, I found these processes to be comparable and decided dental care was as important to one's health as any other part of the body.

"Yes, I am very happy to have had the work done and I would repeat the decision.

"Now at age 73, I am smiling – I can eat apples, carrots, and celery as easily as I can do bananas. It makes me feel so healthy."

That's what the oral-systemic connection is all about. Better dental health leading to better overall health and a preferred quality of life.

---

1 American Heart Association, Inflammation, heart disease and stroke: The role of C-reactive protein, http://www.americanheart.org/presenter.jhtml?identifier=4648, accessed 1/09/08

2 Ibid.

3 Ibid.

4 Ibid.

5 Cushman M, Arnold A, et. al., C-reactive protein and the 10-year incidence of coronary heart disease in older men and women: The cardiovascular health study, Circulation, 2005;1 12:25-31

6 Cook NR, Buring JE, et. al., The effect of including C-reactive protein in cardiovascular risk prediction models for women, Annals of Internal Medicine, Vol. 145 Issue 1, P 21-29, 4 July 2006

7 American Periodontal Association, Periodontal disease, C-reactive protein and overall health, http://www.perio.org/consumer/happy-heart.htm

8 UC Davis study identifies C-reactive protein as cause of blood clot formation, http://www.ucdmc.ucdavis.edu/news/CRP_study.html, accessed 1/10/08

9 Devaraj S et. al., Univ. of California, Davis Medical Center, C-reactive protein increases plasminogen activator inhibitor-1 expression and activity in human aortic endothelial cells, American Heart Assoc. Journal Circulation, 2003;107:398-404

10 Ridker PM, High-sensitivity C-reactive protein – potential adjunct for global risk assessment in the primary prevention of cardiovascular disease, Circulation, 2001;103:1813

11 Study Dismisses Protein's Role in Heart Disease, New York Times, July 11, 2009, accessed online, September 16, 2009

12 Koenig et. al., C-reactive protein, a sensitive marker of inflammation, predicts future risk of coronary heart disease in initially healthy middle-aged men, Circulation, 1999;99:237-242

13 Mahmud A, et. al., Arterial stiffness is related to systemic inflammation in essential hypertension, Hypertension, 2005;46:1118

14 Kullo JJ, et. al., C-reactive protein is related to arterial wave reflection and stiffness in asymptomatic subjects from the community, American Journal of Hypertension, Volume 18, Issue 8, August 2005, pages 1123-1129

15 Pepys MB, Hirschfield GM, et. al., Targeting C-reactive protein for the treatment of cardiovascular disease, Nature, 440, 1217-1221 (27 April 2006)

16 Nissen SE, et. al., Statin therapy, LDL cholesterol, C-reactive protein, and coronary artery disease, New England Journal of Medicine 352:29-38, January 6, 2005 Number 1

17 Sesso HD, Buring JE, et. al., C-reactive protein and the risk of developing hypertension, Journal of the American Medical Association, 2003;290:2945-2951

18 Blake GJ, Rifal N, et. al., Blood pressure, C-reactive protein and risk of future cardiovascular events, Circulation, 2003 ;108 :2993

19 Johns Hopkins, Inflammation marker predicts colon cancer, Journal of the American Medical Association, Feb. 4, 2004, http://www.hopkinsmedicine.org/Press_releases/2004/02_10_04.html

20 Ranjit N, Diez-Roux A, et. al, Psychosocial factors and inflammation in the multiethnic study of atherosclerosis, Archives of Internal Medicine, 2007 ;167:174-181

21 Mattila K, Vesanen M, et. al., Effect of treating periodontitis on C-reactive protein levels : a pilot study, BMC Infectious Diseases, 2002, 2 :30

22 Loos BG, Craandijk J, et. al., Elevation of systemic markers related to cardiovascular diseases in the peripheral blood of periodontitis patients, Journal of Periodontology, October 2000, Vol. 71 No. 10, pages 1528-1534

23 University of North Carolina at Chapel Hill, New research finds link between gum disease, acute heart attacks, UNC News Service, http://www.unc.edu/news/archives/nov00/deliar111300.htm

24 Grossi S, Periodontal therapy lowers levels of heart disease inflammation markers, American Dental Association news release, http://www.ada.org/prof/rsources/pubs/adanews/adanewsarticle.asp?articleid=841

25 Carroll MF, Schade DS, Timing of antioxidant vitamin ingestion alters postprandial proatherogenic serum markers, Circulation, 2003;108:24

26 American Heart Association, AHA/CDC panel issues recommendations on CRP testing, Journal Report 01/28/2003, http://www.americanheart.org/presenter.jhtml?identifier=3007984, accessed 1/12/08

27 Ibid.

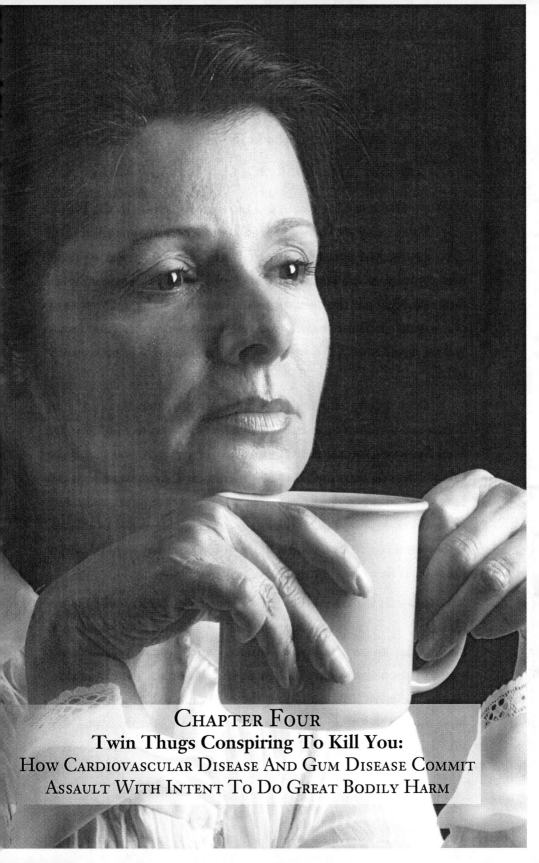

CHAPTER FOUR
Twin Thugs Conspiring To Kill You:
How Cardiovascular Disease And Gum Disease Commit
Assault With Intent To Do Great Bodily Harm

CHAPTER 4
Twin Thugs Conspiring To Kill You
How Cardiovascular Disease and Gum Disease Commit Assault With Intent To Do Great Bodily Harm

Two of the leading causes of death among adults in the United States today are heart attack and stroke. Nearly one-third of all deaths, 32.6 percent to be exact[1], are caused by these two thieves who conspire to rob you of years of productive life. These are stark facts that highlight the need for more Americans to be aware of these oral – systemic connections so you can prevent or reverse gum disease and the devastation it can wreak on your health as well as your quality of life.

We've briefly explored the inflammation link between gum disease and cardiovascular disease. There is another direct link that has been discovered by relatively recent scientific research, and that is the role of infection deep in the arteries. Combined, these two effects can beat up on your body mercilessly. They are twin thugs that, at the very least, will cause you pain. At their worst, they could scheme to kill you. If they were people, there isn't a judge in the land that wouldn't throw the book at them and put them away for life.

Let's start with the verified links between oral health and these terrible two. The connection between heart disease and poor periodontal health is no longer in dispute. In fact, dental health is significantly worse in people who have had an acute heart attack than in healthy people.[2] Researchers examining the relationship between coronary heart disease and poor dental health in middle-aged men found that this linkage was a strong one all by itself, without even considering diseases like diabetes, lifestyle factors such as smoking and other cardiovascular risks they investigated.[3]

Other studies have even quantified the connection. A British study showed that poor oral hygiene and gum disease both increased the risk of coronary heart disease by 25 percent. The risk was 72 percent higher among younger men under the age of 50.[4] Researchers determined that people who have markers for periodontal disease in their bloodstream ran a risk of heart attack that was two to four times higher than those who didn't have gum disease.[5]

Similarly, the correlation between periodontal disease and other cardiovascular events is now very strong. One study found that people who have periodontal disease are nearly twice as like to also have coronary artery disease than people who don't have gum disease. The same research team examined gum disease as a potential cause or at least a risk factor for stroke. They found that people who had an acute stroke caused by a blockage in the blood supply to the brain were more likely to have an oral infection compared with healthy people.[6]

Perhaps their lives could have been extended, and they could have lived more comfortably and actively, if only they had been able to have their gum disease diagnosed and treated.

Can Gum Disease Harden Your Arteries? Unfortunately, Yes.

Medical experts once thought that atherosclerosis – commonly called hardening of the arteries – was due to the build-up of fatty plaques that happened only because of high cholesterol. Later, when the inflammation effect was discovered, some experts believed that this was the primary cause. A more realistic view today is that it's not just one or the other, but the result of both disorders.[7] In an illustration of how these two forces work together, one study found that some types of plaques are ruptured by the inflammation response. Then, blood clots form over the ruptures and can block arteries, leading to heart attack or stroke, depending on where the blockage occurs.[8]

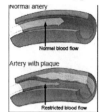

Another inflammation-related factor that ties gum disease to cardiovascular disease was discovered by researchers in Scotland. They found that inflammation from periodontal disease can increase levels of fibrinogen and white blood cells. Fibrinogen is a protein that forms the basis of most clots. White blood cells are a first line of defense against inflammation and play a major role in atherosclerosis. So, as blood levels of these two agents rise as a result of the inflammation, the risk of heart attack may also increase.[9]

Yet another link between gum disease and increased risk of cardiac events was found by examining the associations between deep periodontal pockets and abnormalities in electrocardiograph readings. The researchers concluded that elevated levels of the inflammatory compounds that accompany gum disease cause significant changes in the lesions that lead to hardening of the arteries, heightening the potential for a serious and possibly catastrophic heart attack.[10]

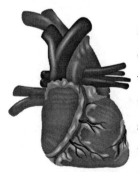

Signs of systemic inflammation are also found in people who have a condition known as degenerative aortic valve stenosis.[11] The aortic valve allows blood to flow from the left ventricle, the lower chamber of the heart, into the aorta and then on through the circulatory system. In this condition, the valve gets clogged and blocks the blood flow. As this valve narrows, the pressure builds up in the left ventricle. The heart works harder to pump against the increased pressure, and the ventricle becomes thicker. That leaves less room for blood to be pumped, which decreases the blood flow even further. Blood may back up into the lungs and fail to reach your brain and the rest of your body with replenishing oxygen and nutrients. Chest pain, shortness of breath, lightheadedness and fainting are common symptoms as this potentially catastrophic scenario unfolds. Of course, a potential complication is heart failure.[12]

The extent of inflammation is even related to how quickly this clogging will progress. Researchers studied men who had this condition in their aorta and classified them into two groups – slow progressors and rapid progressors. Which group they fell into depended on how slowly or quickly their valve continued to plug up, and how much the blood flow through the valve had slowed. After six months, the rapid progressors had significantly higher blood levels of C-reactive protein, the marker that health care professionals use to measure the amount of inflammation present in your body.[13]

Repairing or replacing the valve through surgery has been the preferred treatment. When this valve in the aorta is replaced, other researchers found the blood levels of inflammation markers had decreased six months after surgery compared with pre-surgical levels. Their observations add further weight to the evidence suggesting that aortic clogging is an inflammatory disease.[14]

A New Scientific View: Oral Bacteria May Cause Cardiovascular Disease

Now, research tells us about another culprit who has joined this infamous company of arterial attackers – bacteria from periodontal disease. Hundreds of different types and strains of bacteria are found in the mouth. Don't be alarmed – this isn't necessarily bad, because there are actually some good bacteria. On the other hand, some of these bacteria in your mouth are considered pathogens, infectious organisms that either cause disease or help it develop.

Scientists at the University of Buffalo recently reported that they'd identified two oral pathogens – *Tannerella Forsynthesis* and *Preventell Intermedia* – that are associated with an increased risk for heart attack. However, that same study concluded that ultimately the total number of germs in your mouth has the greatest effect on increasing your odds for heart attack – not just these two pathogens[15].

And, the American Heart Association has identified gum disease as one of the major chronic infections that put you at higher risk for atherosclerosis and coronary heart disease later in life.[16] In fact, one of the main precepts of current periodontal medicine is that oral infection causes a chronic inflammatory burden on the body's entire system. It's based in part on evidence that oral pathogens have evolved the capacity to directly invade tissues throughout the system, triggering inflammatory events that have consequences for other organs and systems.[17]

One of the most common pathogens in periodontal disease is named *Porphyromonous gingivalis,* P. gingivalis for short. While some people who have otherwise good oral health do have P. gingivalis in their mouth, if you have periodontal disease the risk of being infected with this pathogen is more than 11 times greater.[18]

Here's what I find really scary about P. gingivalis and the risk of cardiovascular disease. Once established in your mouth, this bacteria can find its way into your cardiovascular system. Very specific and sensitive scientific testing has

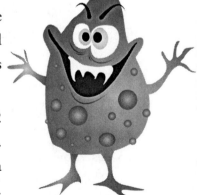

P. gingivalis

actually found its DNA in the tissue of the aorta.19 It shouldn't be there, but once it finds its way from gum tissue into the bloodstream it should be little surprise that it could make itself at home almost anywhere in the body. Exactly what does it do when it gets into the blood and lodges itself in the aorta? We don't know everything yet, but it's certain that it can be up to no good, and the simple fact that it's there is not good news.

What we do know about periodontal bacteria in the bloodstream is that they also find their way into the artery-clogging plaques, where they are believed to play a role in developing coronary artery disease, or in making it worse.[20]

Researchers think there could be several roles these pathogens may play at different stages in the process of hardening and clogging the arteries. One way is by directly infecting the cells that line the artery walls, which would start the inflammation response cascade we talked about earlier. They may also cause the cells of the arterial wall to unleash even more inflammatory signals than usual. Another possibility is that they could increase plaque build-up by stimulating cells to scavenge more cholesterol out of the blood than they normally would. Yet another risk is that, even without invading the lining of the artery, these bacteria could trigger a chain of events that would result in coagulation leading to a blood clot.[21]

In the last scenario, as the blood clot forms it may destabilize any plaque that is already present on the artery wall.[22] The plaque is actually a swelling that bulges out into the artery itself. Inside, there is an accumulation of white blood cells that have scavenged low-density lipoprotein cholesterol and fatty acids, calcium and some connective tissue. The whole thing is covered by a thin fibrous cap that sits in a high mechanical stress zone caused by the continual expansion and contraction as the heart pumps blood through the artery. Once the vulnerable cap ruptures, the tissue debris in the plaque spills into the bloodstream. Too big to pass through smaller downstream branches, the debris chokes off the blood supply and the surrounding tissue dies.

But the worst effects happen when the blood clot that forms over the ruptured plaque grows to the point that it stops blood flow in the artery itself. These are the major events, the sudden heart attacks and strokes, that are often debilitating and frequently fatal.

Whatever the cause and mode of action, researchers now believe that signs of cardiovascular disease may be the inevitable result of a lifetime of continuously accumulating damage from chronic infectious agents in the bloodstream.[23]

Unfortunately, a contemporary lifestyle that features convenience foods that tend to be loaded with the wrong kinds of dietary fats plays right into this entire process. Researchers have found that high fat diets can cause a hyperinflammatory response to P. gingivalis, which only intensifies this whole cascade of potentially life-threatening events.[24]

Gum Disease and Stroke – Another Deadly Duo

With more than 700,000 strokes in the United States each year, this catastrophic cerebrovascular event is one of the leading causes of death. What many don't realize is that it is also the number one cause of serious long-term disability.[25]

Many refer to stroke as a brain attack, probably because most strokes occur when a clot stops the blood flow to the brain, much as an arterial blockage cuts off circulation to or from the heart. This type of event is called an ischemic stroke. There is another kind of stroke in which a blood vessel breaks and bleeds into the brain. This is termed a hemorrhagic stroke.

Together, they can cause paralysis, cognitive damage that interferes with your ability to think clearly, blindness, emotional problems, and difficulty speaking. In addition to the human side of stroke, it also has a devastating economic effect. According to the National Stroke Association, the annual cost in the U.S. alone is estimated at $43 billion.[26]

Gum disease has emerged in recent research as an important risk factor for ischemic stroke, the kind that involves a blockage that stops blood flow to the brain.[27] The nature and extent of damage the stroke may cause depends on where in the brain it occurs and how wide an area it has deprived of critical nutrients.

One study examined oral infections as a potential cause for stroke. The findings determined that, in fact, people who had been diagnosed with an ischemic stroke were more likely than those in a control group to have gum disease.

Another study that began in the 1960s and followed some participants as long as 24 years, found that periodontal bone loss was associated with stroke, especially among men under age 65[28]. Periodontal bone loss is associated with a history of gum disease. Researchers pointed out that if gum disease caused stroke, it could be an important risk factor to identify, particularly in younger men, but noted that further studies were needed to determine the strength of the association between gum disease and stroke.

A third study found that, in older adults, there is evidence of an association between a history of stroke and the cumulative effects of gum disease.[29]

The carotid arteries, which are located on both sides of your neck and deliver blood flow to and from the brain, can be major sites for ischemic stroke. Gum disease plays a significant role here, too. It has been fingered as a culprit in the development of early atherosclerotic lesions in the carotid arteries.[30] Researchers have also found that people who have gum disease are more likely to have thickened carotid arteries, which can also lead to stroke.[31, 32]

Healthcare Will Never Be the Same – and That's a Good Thing

You may be starting to think that we've strayed somewhat afar from the connections between gum disease and your overall health. I don't blame you – this is a lot of information to digest, especially in the context of all these relatively new concepts.

Let me simplify the gist of its importance with a few more facts that I believe can help you tie it all together and, so to speak, get your mind around it. Just a few more, I promise.

Scientists are starting to look at oral health problems as initial signs of clinical disease, a sort of early warning system that raises red flags about dangerous conditions developing in other parts of your body. They now consider the mouth a port of entry for bacterial infections that not only have the potential, but actually do cause harmful effects to your general health status. These researchers point especially to advanced periodontitis as a risk factor for developing heart disease and stroke.[33]

Because of the widespread incidence of periodontal disease, these connections are getting a lot of medical attention. Remember the NIH estimate that 80 percent of all adults in the United States have some form of gum disease? As many as 30 percent have the more severe periodontitis. Researchers think that because it's so common throughout our population, gum disease may be the factor at the root of a significant proportion of infection-associated risks for heart disease.[34]

Part of that increased risk for heart attack and stroke may be due to an effect discovered by researchers at Virginia Commonwealth University. What they found was that in patients with severe periodontal disease, changes in their blood cholesterol increased a particularly dangerous type of low-density lipoprotein (LDL), what you often hear referred to as the bad form of cholesterol. This specific subclass is called small-dense LDL, which is also associated with a decrease in irritation-fighting agents in people who have severe gum disease.[35]

The scientific activity has even led to using your oral health status as a predictor for heart disease. According to one study, even the presence of common problems in your mouth – including gum disease – is as good a predictor of heart disease as your level of cholesterol, which for years was seen as the gold standard of cardiovascular risk.[36]

And, if you still aren't convinced, consider this. One research team wrote, "The emergence of periodontal infection as a potential risk factor for (cardiovascular disease) is leading to a convergence in oral and medical care that can only benefit the patients and the public health."[37]

That tells me a number of things that will affect your health care – and, ideally, your health – for the foreseeable future. First, we will no longer consider your dental health status separately from your overall health. Second, we will no longer treat your oral health problems as isolated issues that affect only your teeth and gums. And third, physicians and dentists will do a lot more treatment collaboratively as a health care team rather than as individual providers who look at only one piece of the pie.

Treatment Works

The other part of the good news is that even though you may already have gum disease, it doesn't have to mean that you're on an irreversible course that leads you straight into the gaping maw of fatal heart disease or stroke. Far from it, in fact. Here, the good news is that treatment not only works in the sense that it can halt the progression of the inflammation cascade and related periodontitis issues. The truth is that treatment for gum disease can also actually reverse some of these effects. This is one of the reasons why an article in a relatively recent issue of Reader's Digest, while surveying the latest scientific research on gum disease and systemic inflammation, was headlined "How your dentist can safe your life" and suggested that "your dentist may be the most important doctor you see this year."[38]

Some of the most intriguing research in this area was done by Aetna, one of the largest health insurers in the U.S. Their interest, of course, is clearly related to their bottom line – after all, the fewer health care claims they pay the greater their potential earnings on their dental coverage and other health insurance products. The results are instructive for those of us in the medical profession and in the health-care policy field, so you can also assign some very real redeeming social value to what may otherwise appear to be an entirely profit-oriented undertaking. Because costs threaten to continue their steep climb into the foreseeable future, it's an area of substantial importance in public policy for government-funded healthcare. The fact that the study was actually conducted by the Columbia University College of Dental Medicine confers significant scientific objectivity.

The study reviewed 145,000 Aetna members who had continuous coverage for both dental and medical care for a period of at least two years. What they found was that periodontal care apparently has a significant effect on the cost of medical care. Even more substantive is the finding that the earlier the treatment the lower the costs for certain diseases – cardiovascular disease, stroke and diabetes. In fact, the actual cost for medical care for heart disease and diabetes was lower if they received periodontal treatment in the first year of the study. One of the investigators, Associate Professor David A. Albert, DDS observed, "The association between periodontal infection and systemic health has important implications for the treatment and management of patients."[39]

Another study found clear evidence that, in people who have a systemic inflammatory reaction to gum disease, periodontal treatment decreases the C-reactive protein levels. As that inflammation marker drops, the researchers believe the associated health risks also decrease.[40]

Other investigators found that a common periodontal treatment called scaling and root planing, combined with a topical antibiotic gel, can lower CRP levels significantly. The results showed that the CRP levels could actually approach the low-risk mark.[41]

These are some of the reasons why, when I train other dentists, I include every aspect of the interconnectedness of your oral and physical health. When they finish this training, these dentists also know how to work with your physician to make sure that your oral health is considered as a factor in the traditional medical treatment of cardiovascular disease and stroke.

Testimonial - Chad Fleetwood

Dental visits don't have to be a headache.

At one time Chad Fleetwood considered dental visits a headache. Little did he know that his visit to our office would help him cure the headaches that had been a constant disruption in his life – and even improve his sleep!

Chad came to our office because his wife was a patient. He came in for a routine cleaning and I could see that his mouth needed some alignment. At that point I recommended an occlusal equilibration.

Now that's a dental term that sounds scary but the procedure isn't scary at all. It's a manual adjustment of your teeth. And what it does is allow your jaw to function as it was meant to function and your teeth to meet properly.

If it's a simple case, it usually can be done and completed in a short period of time. More complex cases may require more than one appointment. Either way, it doesn't have to hurt. Chad's treatment didn't. In fact he described it as "painless."

Chad simply didn't know that the problems he had with his bite were causing him problems with his health. But I'll let him tell you in his own words about the results:

"The occlusal equilibration has changed my life. My constant headaches are gone and I sleep a lot better than I have ever slept. I used to wake up every morning fatigued. I just thought it would be like that for the rest of my life and now with my dental treatment, that is no longer true."

Many TMJ sufferers have their symptoms relieved by an occlusal equilibration and it's used to treat the slight shifting that sometimes occurs after orthodontia is complete. Once an occlusal equilibration is complete you'll be surprised how much better you'll feel and how much easier it is to chew. Yes, your mouth will feel different, but you'll gradually adjust to the new chewing position of your teeth and I'm confident that you'll like the results!

1 National Vital Statistics Reports, CDC, Deaths: Preliminary Data for 2006, Table B, p. 5, http://www.cdc.gov/nchs/data/nvsr/nvsr56/nvsr56_16.pdf, accessed 6/18/08

2 Mattila KJ, Nieminen MS, et. al., Association between dental health and acute myocardial infarction, British Medical Journal 189 ;298 :779-81

3 Briggs JE, McKeown PP, Angiographically Confirmed Coronary Heart Disease and Periodontal Disease in Middle-Aged Males, Journal Periodontol, 2006.77.1.95

4 DeStefano F, Anda RF, et. al., Dental disease and risk of coronary heart disease and mortality, British Medical Journal 306 :688-691, 1993

5 American Dental Association, Study links gum disease, heart attack risk independent of smoking, news release, www.ada.org/prof/resources/pubs/adanews/adanewsarticle.asp?articleid=939

6 American Academy of Periodontology, Heart disease and stroke, http://www.perio.org/consumer/mbc.heart.htm

7 Steinberg D, Atherogenesis in perspective: Hypercholesterolemia and inflammation as partners in crime, Nature Medicine 8, 1211-1217 (2002)

8 Libby P, Atherosclerosis: The new view, Scientific American, May 2002, p. 50 - 59

9 Kweider M, Lowe GD, et. al., Dental disease, fibrinogen and white cell count ; links with myocardial infarction?, Scottish Medical Journal, 1993 June;38(3):73-4

10 American Dental Association, Deep periodontal pockets linked with ECG abnormalities, news release, www.ada.org/prof/resources/pubs/adanews/adanewsarticle.asp?articleid=956

11 Galante A, Pietroiusti A, et. al., C-reactive protein is increased in patients with degenerative aortic valvular stenosis, Journal of the American College of Cardiology, 2001 ; 38 :1078-1082

12 National Library of Medicine, National Institutes of Health, Aortic stenosis, http://www.nlm.nih.gov/medlineplus/ency/article/000178.htm, accessed 6/18/08

13 Sanchez PL, Santos JL, et. al., Relation of circulating C-reactive protein to progression of aortic valve stenosis, American Journal of Cardiology, 2006, Jan, 1;97(1):90-3. Epub 2005 Nov 10

14 Gerber IL, Stewart RA, et. al., Effect of aortic valve replacement on c-reactive protein in nonrheumatic aortic stenosis, American Journal of Cardiology, 2003, Nov, 1 ;92(9) :1129-32

15 Science Daily, The More Oral Bacteria, The Higher The Risk of Heart Attack, April 2, 2009, accessed at http://www.sciencedaily.com/releases/2009/04/090401101848.htm , September 17, 2009.

16 Healthday News, November 29, 2005 – Spokesman for the American Heart Association confirms the link between Perio and Heart Disease, http://health.yahoo.com/news/141399:_vlt=Ahq5pJAqH2GCLGes3r4j7NX3tMUF

17 Paquette DW, Madianos P, The concept of 'risk' and the emerging discipline of periodontal medicine, The Journal of Contemporary Dental Practice, Vol. 1 No.1, Fall 1999

18 Griffen AL, Becker MR, Lyons SR, Moeschberger ML, Leys EJ, Prevalence of Porphyromonous gingivalis and periodontal health status, Journal of Clinical Microbiology, November 1998, 36;11:3239-3242

19 Stelzel M, Conrads G, et. al., Detection of Porphyromonas gingivalis DNA in aortic tissue by PCR, Journal of Periodontology, 2002, Vol. 73, No. 8, Pages 868-870

20 Harasthy VI, Zambon JJ, et. al., Identification of periodontal pathogens in atheromatous plaques, Journal Periodontol, 2000 Oct ;71(10) :1554-60

21 Fong IW, Am J, Infections and their role in atherosclerotic vascular disease, Journal of the American Dental Association, Vol 133, No suppl_1, 7S-13S

22 Zaremba M, Gorska R, et. al., Evaluation of the incidence of periodontitis-associated bacteria in the atherosclerotic plaque of coronary blood vessels, Journal of Periodontology, 2007, Vol. 78, No. 2, Pages 322-327

23 Herzberg MC, Coagulation and thrombosis in cardiovascular disease: Plausible contributions of infectious agents, Annals of Periodontology, 2001, Vol. 6, No. 1, Pages 16-19

24 Beck JD, Offenbacher S, Periodontitis: a risk factor for coronary heart disease?, Annals of Periodontology, 1998 July;3(1):127-41

25 National Institutes of Health, National Institute of Neurological Disorders and Stroke, What You Need To Know About Stroke, http://www.ninds.nih.gov/disorders/stroke/stroke_needtoknow.htm accessed 6/27/08

26 National Institutes of Health, National Institute of Neurological Disorders and Stroke, Questions and Answers About Stroke, http://www.ninds.nih.gov/disorders/stroke/stroke_backgrounder.htm, accessed 6/27/08

27 Wu T et al., Periodontal Disease and Risk of Cerebrovascular Disease, Archives of Internal Medicine, 2000: 160:2749-2755

28 Medical News Today, History of Periodontitis Linked to Cerebrovascular Disease in Men, July 2, 2009, Accessed online at www.medicalnewstoday.com, September 17, 2009.

29 Lee HJ, Garcia RI, The Association Between Cumulative Periodontal Disease and Stroke History in Older Adults, Journal of Periodontology, 2006, Vol. 77, No. 10, Pages 1744-1754

30 Soder P, Soder B, Early Carotid Atherosclerosis in Subjects with Periodontal Diseases, Stroke, 2005;36:1195

31 American Academy of Neurology 51st Annual Meeting, Toronto, CA, 4/21/99, Periodontal Disease May Increase Risk of Stroke, Mitchell Elkind, MD, Columbia University, New York, http://www.pslgroup.com/dg/f896a.htm

32 American Heart Association, Relationship of Periodontal Disease to Carotid Artery Intima-Media Wall Thickness, http://atvb.ahajournals.org/cgi/content/abstract/atvbaha:21/11/1816

33 Rose LF, Mealey B, Oral care for patients with cardiovascular disease and stroke, Journal of the American Dental Association, Vol. 133, No. suppl_1, 37S-44S

34 Genco R, Offenbacher S, Periodontal disease and cardiovascular disease – epidemiology and possible mechanisms, Journal of the American Dental Association, Vol. 133, No. suppl_1, 14S-22S

35 Virginia Commonwealth University, VCU study suggests new link between severe periodontitis and cardiovascular disease, News release, Dec. 1, 2005, http://www.vcu.edu/uns/Releases/2005/dec/120205.html

36 WebMD, Periodontal disease and heart health, April, 2005, http://www.webmd.com/content/Article/104/107270/htm?printing=true

37 Demmer RT, Desvarlieux M, Periodontal infection and cardiovascular disease – the heart of the matter, JADA, Vol. 137, Oct. 2006, Supplement, Pages 15s-20s

38 Readers Digest, How your dentist can save your life, December, 2005, http://www.rd.com/content/openContent.do?contentId=19804

39 Aetna, Aetna and Columbia announce results from study showing relationship between periodontal treatment and a reduction in the overall cost of care for three chronic conditions, Press release, 3/20/2006, http://www.aetna.com/news/2006/pr_20060317.htm, accessed 6/28/08

40 Mattila K, Vesanen M, Effect of treating periodontitis on C-reactive protein levels, BMC Infect Dis. 2002 Dec 10;2:30

41 Grossi S, et. al., SUNY Buffalo, Periodontal therapy lowers levels of heart disease inflammation markers, ADA News 04/21/2004

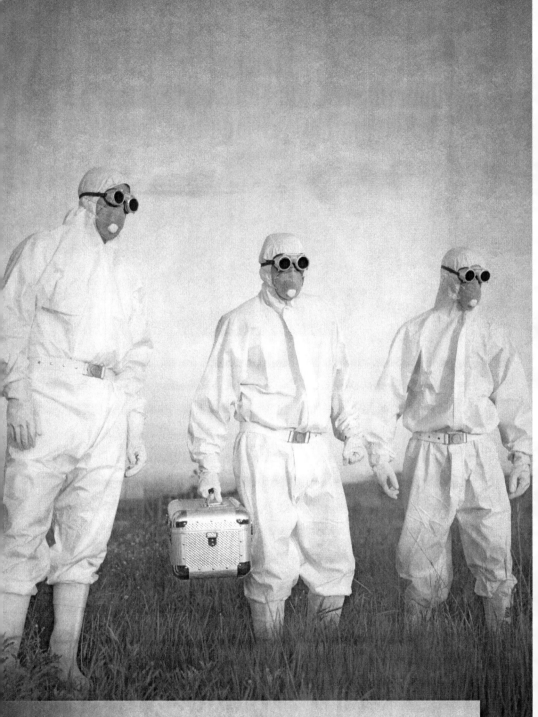

CHAPTER FIVE
Gum Disease, Diabetes And Systemic Inflammation:
A TRIANGLE OF TROUBLE

CHAPTER 5

Gum Disease, Diabetes and Systemic Inflammation: A Triangle of Trouble

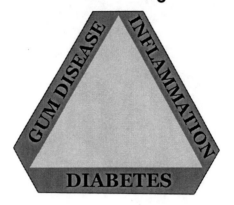

n a previous chapter we briefly touched on the idea that people who have diabetes are at higher risk of developing gum disease. When gum disease occurs in people who have diabetes, it can have a direct effect on their diabetes control. Here we'll describe in more detail about how this vicious cycle works so you know exactly what's at stake and how to prevent a condition that starts in your mouth, worsens your diabetes, and may potentially lead to a life-threatening series of catastrophic health events.

For people who have diabetes periodontal disease is typically worse than in people who don't have diabetes. Research has confirmed that diabetes makes gum disease more severe. Other research indicates that gum disease may be a predictor for developing diabetes, but we're not yet clear whether gum disease treatment can prevent diabetes development. However, that's not a reason to put off treatment, because gum disease left untreated wreaks havoc in your mouth and is linked to other serious diseases. Treating it reduces inflammation levels in the body.

If you have diabetes, your gum disease is likely to include deeper pockets in the gums around the teeth, more loss of bone and more loss of the periodontal ligaments that connect the teeth to the alveolar bone. This is especially true for those whose diabetes is not under control and for those who've had diabetes for many years. The earlier a person develops diabetes and the longer they've had it, especially if they've had problems controlling it, the more susceptible they are to periodontal disease. And, once they get it, the more destructive it is.[1] Illustrating the extent of how much more severe gum disease can be in people with diabetes, one study found that adults with diabetes have four times the alveolar bone loss from periodontal disease as those who don't have diabetes.[2] This is the bone structure that forms the pocket which cradles the tooth to keep it stable and healthy so it can do its job.

If you lose the bone you're well on the way to losing the tooth. Studies show that adults with diabetes have higher rates of tooth loss from gum disease than those without diabetes.[3] In fact, one study showed that toothlessness is 15 times higher in people with diabetes than in people who have not been diagnosed with diabetes.[4] By that time, you're also at much higher risk of systemic interactions with your diabetes that are significantly more serious threats to your health.

Another factor here is the issue of having healthy teeth so they can they can do the job they were designed to do and help you with your daily diet. How so? Well, it's actually quite straightforward.

If you have healthier teeth you can eat a greater variety of foods, both the foods you like and the foods that are good for you which, ideally, are one and the same. Food choices made by people who have poor teeth tend to be softer so they cause less pain during chewing. Softer foods tend to be more dense in calories, fat and refined carbo-hydrates, which are readily converted into high levels of blood glucose.

When you have stronger teeth that give you the option of choosing firm foods, you are better able to follow dietary guidelines and include more fruits and vegetables in your diet. These tend to be lower in calories and fat, and they contain complex carbohydrates. It takes the digestive system more time to convert complex carbs into nutrients that the body can use for energy, and these nutrients enter the bloodstream more slowly.

The chief metabolic result is that you avoid the big spike of blood sugar that you get with foods that are loaded with refined carbohydrates. This often produces a significant improvement in blood glucose control. A frequent side effect is that as these foods are digested more slowly, you are satisfied for a longer period of time after each meal. When you're less hungry, you tend to snack less on high-fat, high refined carb, high-calorie foods that spike your blood glucose and pile on weight.

In fact, I have seen many people with diabetes who get their teeth fixed even start to lose weight, simply because they can eat better foods without oral pain.

If you can keep your diabetes well under control, you have a much better chance of avoiding periodontal diseases. In one national health survey that included thousands of Americans, people with diabetes who kept their blood glucose levels well controlled had no higher risk of developing gum disease than people without diabetes. But those who had diabetes and whose blood sugar was not well controlled had a rate of periodontal disease that was three times higher.[5]

Insulin-dependent diabetes carries a much higher rate of susceptibility to gum disease. One study showed a rate that's nearly six times higher than in those who don't have diabetes.[6]

How does diabetes affect susceptibility to periodontal disease? One way is by reducing the effectiveness of the body's phagocytes.[1,7] These are cells that can engulf and kill other cells, such as the bacteria that are attacking your gums. With your normal defenses lowered by diabetes, the bacteria are free to establish a beachhead and wreak havoc beneath your gum line.

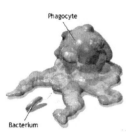

Phagocyte

Bacterium

Another reason why periodontal disease is worse in people with diabetes is the problem of reduced healing capacity. In gum disease, the main effect of this is to lower your ability to repair the tissues that are injured by the inflammation.

This is a particular problem with the periodontal ligaments, which need to be rebuilt with an influx of collagen.6 One of the most common compounds in the entire animal kingdom, collagen makes up about 30 percent of all the proteins in the human body. One medical expert calls it nature's re-bar, comparing it with the steel reinforcement rods that are used in concrete construction. The body's normal response to an injury in connective tissue is to send collagen to the site to repair the defect.[8] If you are already experiencing one of several types of disease states, your body just can't deposit enough collagen to shore up the periodontal ligament, which then continues to fail as gum disease keeps assaulting it.

If you have a health condition that reduces your body's normal healing capacity, that can also make your dental treatment more complex. It's one of the reasons why your dentist needs to know your full history and your current state of health. This is especially true if your dentist needs to do oral surgery to treat your gum disease. Your dentist is almost guaranteed to use non-surgical treatments first, and obviously they won't do any surgery until you're able to heal well. This may take a period of medication with antibiotics and nutraceuticals to restore more of your body's natural ability to heal. We'll go into more detail about this later.

Gum Disease and Diabetes: The Two-Way Street

Researchers have also documented connections that show diabetes and periodontal disease form a two-way street. Just as diabetes makes gum disease worse, gum disease affects how well people with diabetes can control their blood glucose levels. One study showed that people who had diabetes and severe periodontitis had a risk of worsening blood glucose control that was six times higher than those who have diabetes but who didn't have gum disease.[9]

How can periodontal disease affect blood glucose levels? Research so far indicates that it's related to the body's inflammation response. It's clear that both gum disease and diabetes – especially type 2 diabetes – are affected by inflammation. This includes inflammation caused by bacterial infection. In diabetes, bacterial infections that get into the system increase the body's insulin resistance. The cells can't use insulin to transfer glucose out of the blood so the sugar can be burned to provide energy to the cell. As a result, the sugar stays in the blood and raises the blood glucose level.[10]

The exact mechanism creates a circular process of effects that make each other worse. Periodontal diseases often increase blood levels of cells that promote inflammation.[11] These cells are called proinflammatory cytokines. Cytokines are proteins that the body uses to interact or communicate between different types of cells.

People who have diabetes often have high blood concentrations of other cells that take promoting inflammation to an even greater level. These cells are called hyperinflammatory cytokines.

When those two types of inflammation-promoting cells interact due to gum disease in a person who has diabetes, the body responds by releasing even more of the proinflammatory cytokines. The net effect, again, compounds insulin resistance and makes it increasingly difficult to keep blood glucose levels under control and stable.

Periodontal therapy has been found to decrease certain cytokines and increase adiponectin, a protein hormone that moderates metabolic processes including blood glucose regulation.[12]

That's important, because all these additional cells that promote inflammation are also at work to make your gum disease worse. Without treatment, it's like trying to extinguish a fire by dousing it with gasoline.

The Rust Effect: Eating Away At Your Microvascular System

The big life-threatening developments are what we call the macrovascular effects, the damage that is done in the arteries and veins. Now let's consider the issue of what goes on at the microvascular level, in the small, even microscopic, parts of our circulatory system.

This is sort of an off-ramp system, where the blood leaves the arterial express lane then exits the freeway altogether and goes to smaller and smaller surface streets, so to speak, so it can deliver nutrients to individual cells. These pathways include venules, which go between veins and capillaries. Capillaries are the point at which the blood starts exchanging various substances with tissues. A substantial part of the total circulatory activity in the body happens at this level. Capillaries, in turn, connect with arterioles, the smallest part of the system, where only one blood cell squeezes through.

The damage done at this level is precisely what causes a lot of the other problems related to diabetes. These include decreased vision, loss of sensation, impotence and blood pressure problems. This group of effects can cause a significant loss in quality of life by affecting your ability to handle daily living chores, stay active, and keep doing the things you enjoy in life.

Almost all of these are caused by a combination of two factors. First, there is the stiffness in the wall of the blood vessels that we have talked about earlier. Second, there is the rust factor. That's right, rust. It's not a medical term, obviously. It's more of an analogy, and it's very useful because it acts much the same way.

Let's say you leave an old hammer out in the rain and it rusts. You finally find it lying right where you left it, and you pick it up by the head. You notice that the rusty surface is rough and pitted, and the edges of the pits are scratchy, even a little bit sharp.

Now, imagine you have a blood cell that has rust on it. Its surface is scratchy and a little sharp. What happens as that cell wriggles with all its might to work its way through the tiny arterioles? Its sharp edges scratch and scrape at the walls of the arteriole. And, if those walls have lost their elastic qualities due to the hardening process that is triggered by the inflammatory response – which, in turn, was set off by infection by periodontal bacteria – the wall is eventually going to either break or clog. Either outcome is a bad thing.

The rust analogy is appropriate here, too, because your body could end up looking like a rusted-out hulk of an old car from the dinosaur era of automobiles, one that was driven hard and put away wet after too many miles over salted winter roads in the snowbelt. They rusted from the bottom up and inside out. It's not a pretty sight. Even the auto industry, as precarious as it is these days, figured out that undercoating the entire chassis prevents most rust. Unfortunately, protecting your microvascular system from the rust effect just isn't that easy.

Where does the rust come from? It's a process called glycation, which happens when your blood sugar is too high and glucose actually bonds to cells in your blood. When they bond on the outside of the cell, they form the rust with its scratchy, sharp surfaces that wear away at vessel walls.

One of the main problems this causes is called diabetic retinopathy. It's a common complication of diabetes that affects the retina, the membrane that covers the back of the eye and provides the light sensitivity we need to be able to see normally. If this condition is left untreated, it can lead to blindness. Loss of sight is usually preventable if it's diagnosed and treated promptly. As many as 45 percent of all people with diabetes have some level of diabetic retinopathy.13 Damaged fragile blood vessels can leak blood into the center of the eye and blur your vision. It can also lead to increased cataract formation. Frequently there are no symptoms, and there is no pain. Without treatment, you are well on the way to severe vision loss, and possibly total blindness.

Another of these conditions caused by the rust factor is called paresthesia. It's a term for odd sensations of the skin. These strange feelings can range from numbness to burning. They include prickling, tingling, itching or a feeling that something is creeping on your skin. It is usually felt in the extremities – the hands, arms, legs or feet – but can occur in other parts of the body as well. This is the feeling that most of us have had at one time or another when we have sat with our legs crossed for too long. That is actually a temporary paresthesia. The chronic form occurs when nerves are damaged by the microvascular rust effect. While it may not be life-threatening, it's not pleasant and when it flares up it can be so uncomfortable that you just may wish you were dead.

Paresthesia is an early symptom of damage to sensory nerves. It's a warning sign of even worse nerve damage that may be in progress called peripheral neuropathy. Diabetes causes 30 percent of neuropathies, which affect an estimated 20 million Americans. Generally concentrated in the hands and feet, neuropathy is characterized by numbness, tingling, pain and weakness. This indicates serious damage to nerves that send vital control signals that govern your ability to use your limbs for even simple tasks of daily life. Excruciating leg muscle cramps are common for many people who have peripheral neuropathy. Others may lose their ability to feel their feet, which makes walking extremely difficult. There are several more painful and unpleasant symptoms experienced by many people who have diabetes. Some can be helped, but most cannot be cured.[14]

Due to the ever-present ads you see all over TV nowadays, impotence has now become better known by its other name – erectile dysfunction. This condition now affects as many as 45 percent of all men 40 – 69 years old.[15] Yes, there are several causes of impotence, but one of the main ones is any disorder that reduces blood flow in the penis. Diabetes is one of the main physical causes. Combined with the atherosclerosis caused by the inflammation response, the rust effect of glycated blood cells and its damage to nerves, arteries and smooth muscle, as many as 50 percent of men with diabetes experience ED.[16]

We're also seeing a lot of ads on TV now for drugs to treat peripheral artery disease, or PAD. Here, we're basically talking about a blockage in the arteries leading to the extremities, the lower extremities in particular. It's common if you have diabetes to have problems with your feet. Foot sores, ulcers, cramping and pain are frequent in people who have diabetes and a podiatrist often needs to be involved with their care. Just massaging the feet, believe it or not, helps by stimulating blood flow. For those of you who like your feet massaged, there's a good reason for it.

This is an example of another potential complication of unchecked gum disease combined with diabetes, inflammation and the rust effect that can appear to be little more than some periodic discomfort when, in fact, you could actually run the risk of losing your life. One of the best things you can do to help control your diabetes is to get some form of regular daily activity. Many people with diabetes choose walking because it doesn't require any special equipment, you don't have to learn any special techniques, and you can do it at any time. But if you have PAD, it can be difficult and painful to get any exercise. You don't get the exercise, you don't get the metabolic advantages that help control your diabetes.

Now, here's the life-threatening part. The narrowed arteries in the leg and foot choke off the blood supply to the muscles. Deprived of oxygen and nutrients, the muscle cells start screaming for help. You experience this as pain, which can be so severe it's actually debilitating. This effect is called claudication. Some people may only experience it when they walk. When the arterial blockage gets closer to closing off the blood supply altogether, it's even painful when you are at rest.

The next step is that the tissue below the blockage starts to die. As the cells die, ulcers develop. Finally, it progresses to gangrene. Bacteria invade, infection develops and can threaten to spread throughout your bloodstream. The decaying tissue is putrid and painful. The result is, frequently, amputation. Unfortunately, it is not unusual for this tragic chain of events to cause death.

Monitor Your Rust Levels

Before even examining your mouth, if your dentist knows you have diabetes your dentist should ask you about you're A1C level. So, okay, what's an A1C level? And what does it have to do with gum disease, the rust factor, and the rest of your physical health?

The rust factor is my term for a condition called glycated hemoglobin. That's where there's too much glucose in your bloodstream and the sugars begin to attach themselves to red blood cells. That's glycation.

The blood cells that have molecules of glucose attached are called glycated hemoglobin. These are what I call the rust cells. Because they have the extra sugar molecules attached to the outside of their cell wall, they can't smoothly squeeze through the tiny microvascular parts of your circulatory system to deliver nutrients to the tissue cells throughout your body.

But they are pushed through these microscopic arterioles anyway, because the heart continues working harder and harder to pulse the blood to its destination points. Picture a blood cell with its scaly appendages of sugar molecules as it is forced through the miniscule veins, scratching the daylights out of the arterial wall, and you'll have an idea of what's going on. Then, when the glycated blood cell gets to the tissue cell where it's supposed to deliver its nutrients, it breaks the cell wall and actually damages the tissue it was supposed to replenish.

As this process goes on billions of times in vital locations throughout critical organs and tissues all over your body, the cell destruction mounts and continues to compound with every beat of your overworking heart.

The result is the microvascular devastation we talked about earlier, leading to such drastic health effects as blindness, amputation, kidney failure, heart attack and stroke.

Now, here's the importance of your A1C level. That's the way we measure your long-term blood glucose levels. And here are the numbers you need to know. An A1C level of 4 to 6 is normal. A level of 6 to 7 is considered prediabetes. A reading above 7 indicates you have diabetes status.

I say that we think of this as your long-term blood glucose level because it indicates the average of your blood sugar over the past 90 days. Here's why. When the glucose molecules attach themselves to a blood cell, they never leave. That blood cell will be glycated for the rest of its life, or about 90 days. So, by measuring the glycated blood cells, we can see an average of your blood glucose levels for the past three months.

How is this different from the glucose level you see in your daily self-monitoring blood glucose test? That level tells you what the glucose content of your blood is at the moment. You know from your own experience that it goes up and down continually, ideally in an acceptable range. If it gets higher, more cells will become glycated.

Remember that these cells are like the 'What happens in Vegas stays in Vegas' concept – once they're glycated they stay glycated. So if we measure glycated hemoglobin every 90 days, we'll get the average of those ups and downs over the longer term. Too bad there's no quick and easy way to get them to just 'stay in Vegas', so to speak.

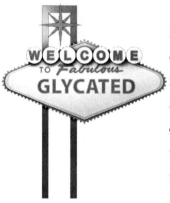

The importance of knowing this number is underscored by every responsible health care organization that is involved with diabetes. In fact, the U.S. Department of Health and Human Services has published thousands of brochures encouraging people who have diabetes to know their blood sugar numbers. The first number they address is your A1C level.[17]

There's an easy way to translate your A1C number so you can relate it to your self-monitoring number. Normal blood glucose is in the range of 90 to 120. That indicates the amount of sugar in milligrams per deciliter of blood. A deciliter is one-tenth of a liter, or about 3.4 ounces. That's just a rate that is useful for lab measurement. A normal person has about five liters of blood in their body.

When I train DentistryForDiabetics® doctors as specialists in providing dental care to people with diabetes, one of the learning tools I use is an illustration of about how much glucose is normally in your bloodstream. I pass out those little packets of sugar that restaurants often give customers for their coffee. That's about five grams of sugar. If you have five grams of sugar in five liters of 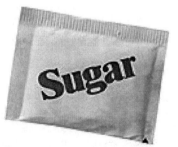 blood, that's 100 milligrams per deciliter. Don't worry if the math gives you fits, just think of it in terms that it's about the same amount that's in the bloodstream of someone who does not have diabetes.

Now, as your A1C number goes up by one, that indicates a rise of about 35 milligrams per deciliter more sugar in your blood.[18] So, for example, let's start with an A1C level of 7, which denotes diabetes. The corresponding reading for that in your self-testing will be 170. If your A1C level rises to 8, your blood glucose level is 205. At an A1C of 9, it's 240. At 10, it's 275, and so on.

I once had a new patient who wanted implants, but after only one look in his mouth I could tell he had diabetes. He said his A1C was 13. That meant he had a blood glucose level of about 380! His metabolic control was absolutely gone, and he had an abundance of glycated hemoglobin cells wreaking havoc throughout his body. He may not have known it yet, but at that rate it likely wouldn't have been long before he would begin experiencing some serious symptoms.

Remember that destructive cycle of inflammation that is triggered by periodontal disease and worsened by diabetes? Part of the damage that occurs is alveolar bone loss. Within six weeks that fellow would certainly have had significant bone loss, and there isn't a dentist in the world who would attempt implants until his diabetes was back under control.

I know we went through some highlights earlier about a few of the scary diseases caused by an out-of-control rust factor. But I absolutely have to top it off with a little more about A1C and health risks. Here is a statistic that is really ugly. Only 30 percent of adults with type 2 diabetes have achieved a level of A1C less than 7.

Just how much of a health risk does a high A1C level represent? The U.S. Agency for Healthcare Research and Quality (AHRQ) wanted to see if they could quantify the relationship between glycation and disease. What they found was that people with diabetes who had A1C readings in the highest categories studied ran much greater risks for certain types of retinopathy, which damages the tiny vessels in your retina. How much greater risk? Up to 13 times higher than people who were in the lowest A1C category.[19]

The agency also found that the risk of potentially fatal coronary artery disease was as much as 70 percent higher. Also, the risk of peripheral artery disease was as much as six times higher.[20]

Other research has found that high levels of A1C are tied to increased risk of death related to atherosclerosis in the carotid artery. The study found that this higher risk is present even with modestly elevated A1C levels.[21]

The good news is that you can keep your A1C level in check and significantly reduce your risk of serious and damaging complications. The AHRQ study found that intensive therapy helped people with diabetes reduce their A1C levels and maintain them at about 7. Their risks went down substantially compared with those who were treated with more conventional therapy and whose A1C leveled off at about 9.[22]

In general, for every point you can lower your A1C level, the risk of microvascular complications associated with diabetes goes down by as much as 37 percent.[23] That's a huge difference.

If you keep your glucose level under tight control and your dental health in good shape, you can probably live a pretty normal life. Tight glycemic control is really important. We frequently see the negative results when the wheels come off the metabolic control. I can't count the number of times that a patient who has been diagnosed as having diabetes and who usually does really well at managing their blood glucose. Then it happens – they come in for normal maintenance, I take one look in their mouth and ask simply, "What happened?" I already know the answer – they lost control of their blood glucose, their A1C level is sky high, and they're paying the price with much worse oral health and rust effect damage occurring throughout their body.

In fact, periodontal care has been shown to improve glycemic control. When blood glucose was measured at three and six months after basic non-surgical periodontal treatment, patients who had diabetes showed improved metabolic control with lower A1C levels.[24]

When dentists use antimicrobial therapy to attack the bacterial infections that have taken hold in gum disease, the results of one research project demonstrated that the treatment also improves metabolic control in people who have diabetes by reducing A1C levels.[25]

Because treatment of gum disease is so effective in reducing A1C levels, experts now consider control of periodontal infection as an important part of the overall management of diabetes.[26]

If You Haven't Been Diagnosed, Take The Diabetes Risk Test

You could have diabetes and not even know it. In fact, nearly a third of those who have diabetes living in the United States today aren't aware that they have the disease.

The American Diabetes Association has a handy tool for find out what risk you run for developing type 2 diabetes.

Answer just seven quick questions and you'll get an immediate answer. If you're at medium to high risk of developing diabetes, you'll also get some general suggestions for ways to reduce your risk.

The test is available on the Web at http://diabetes.org/risk-test.jsp.

A1C Testing: When and How

Now that you know a little about A1C levels, what they measure, and how important they can be, the question is should you have your A1C level tested?

The answer is an absolute, positive resounding yes. Not for the purpose of diagnosing whether you have diabetes. The fasting plasma glucose test is still the preferred method for diagnosis for many.

For regular monitoring of your long-term average blood glucose, the A1C test is the gold standard.

How often should you test your A1C level? The American Diabetes Association Standards of Care, which provide guidelines for medical professionals who treat people who have diabetes, recommends different testing intervals for patients depending on how stable they are able to maintain their blood sugar control.[27]

If you are meeting your treatment goals and your glycemic control is fairly stable, the ADA recommends testing at least twice a year. If you are not meeting your glycemic goals, or if your therapy has changed significantly, you should get your A1C tested every three months.[28]

A1C testing can be done without a period of fasting, and many health care professionals have the equipment to do a test right in their office using the finger stick method.[29] You can wait for the results and discuss them with your dentist or physician right away. This is referred to as point-of-care testing, which allows you and your health care professional to adjust your treatment as necessary, right on the spot.

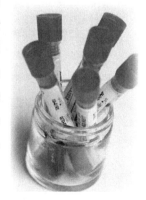

Now there's even a home test for A1C.[30] It is an over-the-counter test, which means that you can buy it without a prescription, although some drug store chains only offer it online. The manufacturer says it will deliver results in just five minutes. The FDA says the test provides results that are comparable to the results of tests done by medical professionals. You may want to discuss this option with your dentist or physician.

What kind of A1C goal should you aim for? It's clear that lowering your A1C level to an average of around 7 reduces microvascular health risks, and may even reduce the risk of macrovascular disease. So, for most adults with diabetes, the initial goal should be 7.[31]

Obviously, lower is better. Scientific studies suggest that lowering A1C from 7 into the normal range continues to provide additional benefits of risk reduction, even though they are smaller than the benefits of reaching the 7 range initially. The closer you can get to normal, right around the 6 range, the more you will be able to prevent potential health complications.[32]

Some people who have diabetes find that reaching that level is difficult without going too far the other way and experiencing hypoglycemia, or low blood sugar. That carries its own set of potential risks. If you have a history of severe hypoglycemia or other associated conditions, your dentist or physician may relax the goals a bit. That's especially true if you have had diabetes for many years and you have few microvascular complications.[33]

The Good News

Lest you may begin to think that this doesn't sound much like a significant health threat, keep in mind the possibility that this cytokine interaction may be going on without any symptoms that are obvious to you, other than an increase in blood glucose. Recall that we pointed out earlier that you may have periodontal disease without any symptoms at all. So you may watch your blood glucose continue to rise, and go to your physician to check it out. Your doctor may not look for an oral connection and may be vexed by not being able to nail down any other cause, but may adjust your insulin or oral medication in response so that your blood glucose remains in control. And you may think to yourself, "Well, I guess my diabetes is just getting worse."

That's true, it is getting worse. But in this case, there's a very good reason for that, and it's one that is readily treated. There is plenty of evidence in the scientific literature showing that treating gum disease can rapidly reverse rising blood glucose. One study found that people with diabetes experienced a clinically significant improvement in their periodontal disease after basic non-surgical treatment.[34] Just three months later, their diabetes had also improved and six months later they were still keeping it better controlled.

Another study showed that treatment to reduce the number of bacteria in the pockets that form around your teeth from gum disease also significantly improved control of diabetes. The researchers said this is probably due to reducing the inflammatory response, which also lowers your body's insulin resistance, which means that your cells can successfully transfer glucose from your bloodstream so it can be used for energy.[35] The net result is that the glucose transferred into tissue cells for energy is no longer in your bloodstream, so your blood sugar levels fall.

Other researchers confirmed a different effect of improved blood glucose levels, and said that controlling periodontal infections is an important part of the overall management of diabetes.[36]

The health risks of periodontal disease combined with diabetes are more than just a nuisance that will result in another trip to your dentist and your physician. They can actually threaten your life.

There is a significant amount of evidence that gum disease may contribute to higher rates of premature death for people who have diabetes.[37] In fact, some researchers have determined that periodontal disease is a reliable predictor of higher death rates among diabetes patients.[38] One study found that people with diabetes who have severe periodontal disease had a death rate of 28.4 percent, while those with little or no gum disease had a death rate of 3.7 percent.[39]

In addition to overall higher death rates, deaths due to certain specific diseases are also higher in people with diabetes who also have periodontal disease. The National Institute of Diabetes and Kidney disease found that gum disease for diabetes patients is a predictor for death from heart disease due to an arterial blockage, as well as for death from kidney disease due to diabetes.[40] Compared with groups who had no gum disease, or even mild to moderate periodontal disease, those who had diabetes and severe periodontal disease ran a risk of death that was more than three times higher. The study found that when the gums pull away from the teeth due to severe periodontal disease, bacteria can enter the bloodstream and affect the heart and kidney.[41]

The risk of stroke is also higher, due to hardening of the arteries that can happen at a much faster rate when you have both diabetes and gum disease[42] and possibly to the bone loss that occurs from gum disease.[43]

The tragedy is that many people with diabetes aren't able to keep their blood glucose under control and experience all the negative health effects that go along with that, when a simple dental checkup could stem the rising tide, or even reverse it.

Patient Profile - William Hanes

"It's one of the best things I have ever done."

We have known Bill Hanes for many years. A regular patient, he had some bridgework and a couple of implants done but had been putting off some needed cosmetic work. Finally, he decided to go ahead with it. Then events took an unexpected turn. Here's Bill's story in his own words.

"At one of my earlier regular checkups, the hygienist noticed that one of my bottom teeth was loose. I hadn't noticed it and it wasn't bothering me so I didn't do anything about it. But it was gradually getting looser and looser. Eventually, I wouldn't bite into anything hard like an apple for fear that I'd lose it. I started getting quite concerned that it needed support so it wouldn't get worse.

"My bottom teeth were sort of livable, but with the tooth getting loose I had to do something about that. A couple of the teeth had some enamel that was getting weak and chipping. I also decided I wanted my teeth to look better, so I went ahead with a restoration.

"My new teeth are great. Looking back, I should have done it a long time ago. My family have all commented on how good they look now.

"I noticed I was getting more and more fatigued, but I just chalked it up to aging. Then I started having to go to the bathroom constantly. My sister finally talked me into seeing the doctor. That's when I was diagnosed as having diabetes.

"As soon as Dr. Martin found out about my diagnosis, he recorded all my medications and my medical status. He asked me about my A1C levels, which were a little high. Now, he factors my diabetes into my dental treatment.

"He told me to be more aware of gum problems and to stay on top of brushing and cleaning to keep my oral health in good shape. Overall, I learned that I need to be more careful with my dental hygiene.

"Now, I also take vitamins and antioxidant supplements which I understand can help people who have diabetes maintain good dental health.

"Looking back, I think I probably had diabetes for a long time but was undiagnosed because I wasn't really sick.

"It is great to have a dentist who knows so much about oral health care for people with diabetes. Instead of having a checkup every six months, I now go every four months so if any problem develops we can deal with it right away.

"Everything's great so far. I'm doing quite well. And I don't worry about that loose tooth anymore.

"I love my new teeth. I wish I had done it a lot earlier. People say I look great. It's one of the best things I've ever done.

Bill's experience is so typical of people whose diabetes hasn't been diagnosed. Hindsight is always perfect, but I wish we had known about some of Bill's other symptoms like his fatigue and constant need to go to the bathroom. Perhaps we could have helped him and his physician diagnose the diabetes earlier.

Please feel free to share physical symptoms with your dentist. Your physical health and your oral health are so intertwined that you really can't separate the two. And it's better to be safe than to look back and wonder. There's absolutely nothing to lose by checking out a symptom. The worst that can happen is you identify a problem earlier than if you hadn't said anything. And, the earlier it's diagnosed the earlier you can begin treatment to halt or even reverse any damage.

When you entrust your care to a DentistryForDiabetics® doctor, you can be sure that you're seeing an elite professional who has in-depth knowledge about meeting the unique oral and physical health needs of people with diabetes.

1Grant-Theule DA, Periodontal disease, diabetes, and immune response: a review of current concepts, J West Soc Periodontol Periodontal Abstr, 1996;44(3):69-77

2 Taylor GW, Burt BA, Becker MP, et al. Non-insulin dependent diabetes mellitus and alveolar bone loss progression over 2 years. J Periodontol 1998;69(1):76-83

3 Diabetes Monitor, Prevention and detection of periodontal disease in diabetics, www.diabetesmonitor.com/b285.htm, accessed 12/31/07

4 Ibid.

5 Tsai C, Hayes C, Taylor GW. Glycemic control of type 2 diabetes and severe periodontal disease in the US adult population. Community Dent Oral Epidemiol 2002;30(3):182-92

6 Loe H, Genco RJ, Oral complications in diabetes, http://diabetes.niddk.nih.gov/dm/pubs/america/pdf/chapter23.pdf, accessed 12/31/07

7 Ibid.

8 Diegelmann RF, Collagen metabolism, http://www.medscape.com/viewarticle/423231, accessed 12/31/07

9 Taylor GW, Burt BA, Becker MP, et al. Severe periodontitis and risk for poor glycemic control in patients with non-insulin-dependent diabetes mellitus. J Periodontol 1996;67(supplement 10):1085-93

10 Yki-Jarvinen H, Sammalkorpi K, Koivisto VA, Nikkila EA. Severity, duration and mechanisms of insulin resistance during acute infections. J Clin Endocrinol Metab 1989;69(2):317-23

11 Loos BG, Craandiji J, Hoek FJ, Wertheim-van Dillen PME, van der Velden U. Elevation of systemic markers related to cardiovascular diseases in the peripheral blood of periodontal patients. J Periodontol 2000;71(10):1528-34

12 American Academy of Periodontology, Journal of Periodontology Online, Adipokines and Inflammatory Mediators Following Initial Periodontal Treatment in Type 2

Diabetic Chronic Periodontitits Patients, http://www.japonline.org/doi/abs/10.1902/jop.2009.090267, accessed September 16, 2009.

13 National Eye Institute, National Institutes of Health, Diabetic retinopathy resource guide, http://www.nei.nih.gov/health/diabetic/retinopathy.asp, accessed 1/16/08

14 The Neuropathy Association, About Peripheral Neuropathy: Facts, http://www.neuropathy.org/site/PageServer?pagename=About_Facts, accessed 5/6/08

15 National Kidney and Urologic Diseases Information Clearinghouse, National Institutes of Health, Kidney and urologic diseases statistics for the United States, http://kidney.niddk.nih.gov/kudiseases/pubs/kustats/#up, accessed 1/16/08

16 National Kidney and Urologic Diseases Information Clearinghouse, National Institutes of Health, Erectile dysfunction, http://kidney.niddk.nih.gov/kudiseases/pubs/impotence/index.htm, accessed 1/16/08

17 U.S. Department of Health and Human Services, National Diabetes Education Program, If you have diabetes . . . know your blood sugar numbers!, NIH Publication No. 98-4350, Revised July 2005

18 Ibid.

19 Use of Glycated Hemoglobin and Microalbuminuria in the Monitoring of Diabetes Mellitus. Summary, Evidence Report/Technology Assessment: Number 84. AHRQ Publication No. 03-E048, July 2003. Agency for Healthcare Research and Quality, Rockville, MD. http://www.ahrq.gov/clinic/epcsums/glycasum.htm

20 Ibid.

21 Jorgensen L, Jenssen T, et. al, Glycated hemoglobin level is strongly related to the prevalence of carotid artery plaques with high echogenicity in nondiabetic individuals, Circulation, 2004;110:466-47

22 Ibid.

23 National Institutes of Health and Centers for Disease Control and Prevention, National Diabetes Education Program, Guiding principles for diabetes care: For health care providers, April, 2004

24 Faria-Almeida R, Navarro A, et. al., Clinical and metabolic changes after conventional treatment of type 2 diabetic patients with chronic periodontitis, Journal of Periodontology 2006.050084

25 The effect of antimicrobial periodontal treatment on circulating tumor necrosis factor-alpha and glycated hemoglobin level in patients with type 2 diabetes, J Periodontol 2001;72:774-778

26 Grossi S, et. al., SUNY Buffalo, Treatment of periodontal disease in diabetics reduces glycated hemoglobin, J Periodontaol 1997;68:713-719

27 American Diabetes Association, Executive summary: Standards of medical care in diabetes – 2008, Diabetes Care, 31:S5-S11, 2008

28 Ibid.

29 Bayer HealthCare Diabetes Care, A1C Testing, 0391904 Rev. 4/07

30 MetrikaA1C, http://www.metrika.com/patients-families/overview/, accessed 1/28/08

31 ADA, op. cit.

32 Ibid.

33 Ibid.

34 Faria-Almeida R, Navarro A, et. al., Clinical and metabolic changes after conventional treatment of type 2 diabetic patients with chronic periodontitis, Journal of Periodontology 2006.050084

35 The effect of antimicrobial periodontal treatment on circulating tumor necrosis factor-alpha and glycated hemoglobin level in patiens with type 2 diabetes, J Periodontol 2001;72:774-778

36 Grossi S, et. al., Treatment of periodontal disease in diabetics reduced glycated hemoglobin, J Periodontaol 1997;68:713-719

37 Loe H, Genco RJ, Periodontal disease and mortality in type 2 diabetes, Oral Complications in Diabetes, http://care.diabetesjournals.org/ogi/reprint/28/1/27

38 National Institute of Diabetes and Digestive Kidney Disease, Periodontal disease predicts mortality in diabetics, Diabetes Care 2005;28:27-32

39 Periodontal disease predicts mortality in diabetics, http://www.defeatdiabetes.org/Articles/periodontal1050124.htm

40 ADA news release, Periodontal disease linked to mortality in diabetes patients: study, http://www.ada.org/prof/resources/pubs/adanews/adanewsarticle.asp?articleid=1219

41 ADA news release, Poor oral health puts patients with diabetes at higher risk of death, http://www.ada.org/public/media/releases/o310_release07.asp

42 Friedlander AH, Maeder LA, The prevalence of calcified carotid artery atheromas on the panoramic radiographs of patients with type 2 diabetes mellitus, Oral Surg Oral Med, Oral Pathol, Oral Radiol, Endod 2000:89:420-4

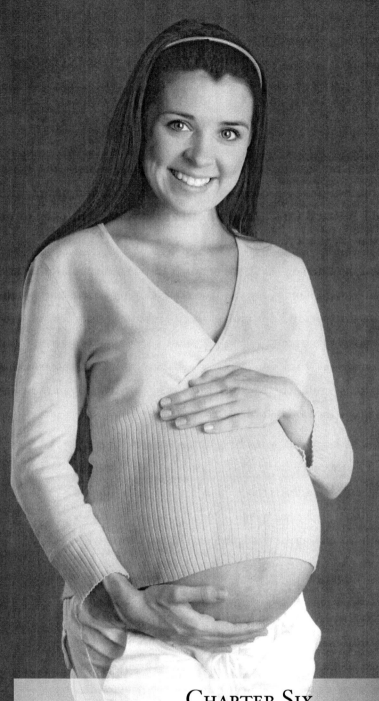

CHAPTER SIX
Oral Health & Pregnancy:
HEALTHY GUMS FOR A HEALTHY BABY

CHAPTER 6
Oral Health & Pregnancy: Healthy Gums For A Healthy Baby

I t's been my experience that very few people – including many in the healthcare professions – associate good oral health with good prenatal care. After all, what do your teeth have to do with your pregnancy?

Yet, the facts are that gum disease can put both the mother and the fetus or the infant at terrible risk of developing serious and potentially life-threatening conditions. It's particularly risky for all concerned when this occurs during pregnancy. As a father of five, I can emphatically say that no parent would even think of intentionally starting their child out in life with having to battle against health threats that start even before birth.

The primary risk posed by gum disease during pregnancy is preterm delivery (PTD) and low birth weight (LBW), but researchers have also linked gum disease to gestational diabetes, which can be a factor in PTD. These studies all suggest that good oral health care is critical before and during pregnancy, to remove as many risk factors for PTD and LBW as possible.

Preterm delivery and low birth weight can threaten the physical health of the baby and the mother, a tragic situation to be sure. Equally tragic is the effect that this has on the emotional health of the entire extended family and its circle of friends. Compounding the angst that can surround what should be a happy event is the fact that, in the case of causes related to periodontal disease, it is largely preventable.

Before we go into the details, let me just say a few words of caution. This is not intended to scare you – it's meant to help you be prepared to deliver the healthy baby you want. It's simple and straight-forward. If you are pregnant, planning a pregnancy or even if you are a woman of childbearing years who may become pregnant, be sure to talk with your dentist. Ideally, you'll do this before you are pregnant so you and your dentist together can make certain your oral health is in great shape so it won't pose any risks to your baby.

Now, here are the facts. The latest statistics show that nearly 13 percent of all births in the United States are preterm. In 2005, that meant that there were more than half a million preterm births.[1] Premature birth is defined as a baby born before the 37th week of pregnancy.2

Premature babies, or preemies, may face numerous health problems. Born before they could go through that spurt of pre-birth weight gain, about eight percent are born with low birth weight, which is considered anything under 2,500 grams, or about five pounds eight ounces. Another one and a half percent are born at very low birth weight – under 1,500 grams or three pounds four ounces.[1]

Because their organs may not have had time to develop fully, preemies typically need a neonatal intensive care unit, where they receive special medical care until their organs and all their systems can work on their own.

Most premature babies can catch up within a year or two, but some aren't so lucky and experience a daily struggle just to survive. Some very serious complications of PTD are, unfortunately, common.[3]

- A heart problem common in preemies is called patent ductus arteriosis. If it isn't treated, it can lead to heart failure,

- A potentially dangerous intestinal problem called necrotizing enterocolitis.

- In babies born before 32 weeks, bleeding in the brain – called intraventricular hemorrhage – can cause brain damage.

- Another common problem in infants born before 32 weeks is called retinopathy of prematurity, an eye problem that in severe cases can cause vision loss unless treated.

- Babies born before 34 weeks may have respiratory distress syndrome, a serious breathing problem.

Obviously, these are not trivial issues that any caring parent would want their child to experience, especially at such an early and vulnerable stage. It's much better to do everything you can before your pregnancy and while you are pregnant so you can delivery a full-term healthy baby. I think it's safe to say that all parents would rather deal with the normal challenges of raising an infant than with serious health risks or, even worse, trying to cope with grief and loss.

The stark facts are, according to some recent data, that preterm delivery is the most frequent cause of infant death in the United States. In a report issued in 2007, the U.S. Department of Health and Human Services said the latest statistics showed that fully 36.5 percent of all infant deaths were due to causes related to preterm delivery. It's even higher for some cultural minorities – nearly half of infant deaths among babies born to non-Hispanic black women, and 41 percent among Puerto Rican women.[4]

Now, obviously, not all infant mortality is related to gum disease. There are far too many causes to go into here. Let's turn now to the links between oral health and a healthy pregnancy.

Infection Is Key

The chief link between periodontal disease, preterm delivery and low birth weight babies can be summed up in a single word: Infection.

Mounting evidence suggests that preterm birth is triggered, or at least contributed to, by a chronic oral infection that leads to an immune reaction. It's the immune response itself that is believed to be the culprit here. It's a bit of a dental mystery whodunit, and here's how it unfolds.

Studies have clearly established the role that infections play in preterm birth. This is especially true for very early preterm birth. We have significantly increased our understanding of the interactions between infection and immunity involving both the mother and the fetus. We now know that bacterial pathogens can cause PTB and LBW either directly or through the immune processes.[5]

Here's how it works. When the body experiences an infection, its white blood cells release proteins called cytokines. These cells come with several different kinds of specialized immune features that boost the body's immune response to the infection. As part of this response in pregnant women, the body releases a cascade of enzymes in both the mother and the fetus that may initiate preterm labor and prematurely rupture the membranes.[6]

Many types of infections have been associated with this phenomenon and the risk for preterm delivery, including periodontal infections. What's particularly interesting to current investigators is findings that suggest some women may have a genetic variation in their reaction to infection that intensifies the body's immune response, placing them and their baby at increased risk for PTB.[7]

An infection during pregnancy may also carry other consequences for the infant beyond the risks of preterm birth and low birth weight. Some types of cytokines that are released in the immune response are also implicated in cerebral palsy in premature babies, as well as depression in mothers.[8]

In fact, relatively recent research has suggested that infection is responsible not only for the preterm birth itself, but also for many of the serious health problems that PTB LBW babies experience, including some of those on that long list of bullet points we just went through. Scientists now believe that new approaches must be developed to prevent prematurity, including some promising ones that focus on preventing or treating infection during pregnancy.[9]

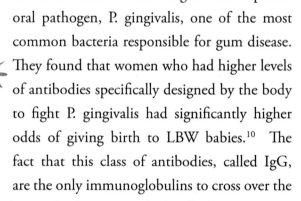

One study has even connected low birth weight with a specific oral pathogen, P. gingivalis, one of the most common bacteria responsible for gum disease. They found that women who had higher levels of antibodies specifically designed by the body to fight P. gingivalis had significantly higher odds of giving birth to LBW babies.[10] The fact that this class of antibodies, called IgG, are the only immunoglobulins to cross over the placenta from the mother to the fetus,11 undoubtedly has important implications for future research into prevention and treatment.

Researchers have also looked at other pathways linking preterm birth and periodontal disease. In one study, investigators examined 48 mothers who delivered preterm low birth weight babies to determine whether there is, indeed, a connection. They measured levels of certain immune-related compounds in the crevices of these mothers' gums. What they discovered was that these fluids contained significantly higher levels of these compounds in the PTB LBW mothers compared with women in a control group.[12]

One of the compounds they found is a certain type of prostaglandin. These are a group of hormone-like substances that play a role in a number of body functions. Among them is controlling inflammation.[13] What inflammation, you ask? Well, remember our earlier discussion about periodontal bacteria that are pathogens and how they cause inflammation – not just locally in the gum, but throughout the body's entire system? Right – that inflammation.

The researchers also found another compound called interleukin. This is a type of protein which has a primary purpose of stimulating the growth of cells that fight off disease.[14]

Another effect of gum disease during pregnancy has to do with something called growth restriction. The full term is intrauterine growth restriction, which refers to a fetus that weighs in at the bottom 10 percent for its age. This can be due to any of several causes, including poor nutrition, congenital abnormalities, genetics or risk factors that the mother may have. It's a condition that increases the risks of complications both during pregnancy and after delivery.[15]

A five-year study called Oral Conditions and Pregnancy, or OCAP, performed full periodontal examinations before the 26th week of pregnancy and again within 48 hours after delivery. The idea was to assess changes in oral health status during the pregnancy, and determine whether there was any association with preterm delivery and growth restriction.

Here's what the OCAP researchers found. The presence of gum disease during the pregnancy and the progression of the disease resulted

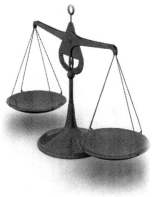

not only in a significantly higher rate of preterm births. It also was associated with a smaller birth weight for the infants' gestational age. In other words, mothers who have gum disease while they're pregnant are not only more likely to deliver prematurely; they're also likely to have a low birth weight baby. And, not only is the baby's birth weight lower than a full-term baby – which could be expected with any preterm delivery – it's also lower than would be expected for a baby delivered at that specific point in the pregnancy.[16]

The Gestational Diabetes – PTD – Gum Disease Risk

Often the increased risk between gum disease and developing gestational diabetes during pregnancy is also associated with other risk factors like smoking or drinking. But a study released in April 2009 by New York University in collaboration with the University of Peradeniya in Sri Lanka[17] found that gum disease by itself increases the chance of developing gestational diabetes, even when other risk factors are absent.

Among the study participants who developed diabetes during their pregnancy, researchers found higher levels of bacteria that cause gum disease as well as greater areas of inflammation. Other risk factors – specifically smoking and drinking – were n the group of participants. More than a third of the women reported bleeding gums when they brushed their teeth. A special test designed for gestational diabetes found that those who had the most bleeding also had the highest blood sugar levels.

Even though gestational diabetes usually disappears after delivery, there is still a substantial risk. Women who develop a high blood sugar count during pregnancy have a bigger risk of PTD and of developing type 2 diabetes later in life. The scientists who investigated these links suggest that women who plan to become pregnant should see their dentist for a thorough checkup and prompt dental care for any signs of problems. Women who are already pregnant should do the same, they said.

A Powerful Argument For Good Dental Care

To me, this finding powerfully underscores the need to factor good oral health care into any prenatal health plan to give your baby the best chance possible to go through a full-term pregnancy and avoid all the potentially debilitating or even fatal complications that accompany preterm delivery and low birth weight and to help you try to avoid the possibility of developing diabetes later in life.

As a chronic infection of your gums and other oral structures that support your teeth, periodontal disease is a destructive inflammatory condition that can readily trigger all the body's immune defenses through an inflammation response cascade that hunts down the inflammation throughout your system so it can be controlled or eliminated. Unfortunately, these same processes also work against your pregnancy by triggering preterm birth.

Here's another way to think about it. Now, keep in mind that this is only my way of interpreting in practical terms what the scientific data to date can tell us and, even though it's based on the science, it's really speculation. I believe this is a natural process of self-preservation designed to protect the host – that's you. The body senses the infection through its powerful inflammation-fighting immune system. It interprets the condition as a potential threat to your life, so it responds by doing everything it can to protect your body, including ending the pregnancy that places major demands on so many organs and, indeed, on your entire system. I realize that, in medical terms, that's a simplistic view but it may also help some people frame in practical terms these mysterious processes that we've really only begun to explain.

The Stakes Are As High As They Can Get

The stakes couldn't be higher. Compared with normal birth weight infants, low birth weight babies are nearly 20 times more likely to die before their first birthday.[10] Babies born to mothers with gestational diabetes may have hypoglycemia, may develop jaundice or may have breathing problems. When you consider the effect periodontal disease can have on preterm birth and gestational diabetes and the complications it adds to a pregnancy, it can be downright frightening.

One team of experts extrapolated the data and suggested that 18 percent of the preterm low birth weight infants born each year may be caused by periodontal disease. That's nearly one-fifth of all PTB LBW births.[18]

Apply that calculation to the 522,913 preterm births for 2005, the latest data available,1 and you arrive at 94,125 infants who potentially could have gone full term. It absolutely stuns me to think that we could prevent that much disease and yes, even death, simply by making certain that expectant mothers have good oral health care.

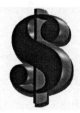 In that same vein, you can also look at the $5.5 billion (yes, that's billion with a great big capital B) that we spend each year in hospital costs to care for preterm low birth weight infants and

calculate a corresponding proportion as related to gum disease.[19] That's about $1 billion! Every year!

I can guarantee that preventing gum disease through good oral health care in women who are pregnant or who are planning a pregnancy would cost only a small fraction of that $1 billion. And the best part is that we would have prevented all that needless human suffering.

So, if we're going to get serious about preventing preterm delivery associated with periodontal disease, and we certainly should, how do we go about it?

Well, the best way is to make certain that all prenatal care involves at minimum an oral health screening. Unfortunately, the national clinical practice guideline for routine prenatal care doesn't even mention oral health or periodontal screening.[20] The thing to keep in mind about these guidelines is that they're developed by medical and professional associations, so they're really voluntary. The problem is getting these professions to recognize and accept the research, include it in the guideline, and disseminate it thoroughly throughout all relevant medical practices.

It's a big job, and believe me, we're trying. The history of these guidelines shows that it takes years to go through this process and actually wind up with a new recommendation getting implemented in individual practices.

What I'm trying to say in a polite, sensitive and politically correct way is that, until this can happen with periodontal screening as a part of routine prenatal care, you're basically on your own. If you're going to get screened for gum disease as a part of conscientiously doing everything you can to have a healthy pregnancy and deliver a full-term healthy baby, you'll have to initiate it yourself to make sure it happens.

Certainly, many dentists will pay special atter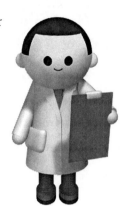 at a routine cleaning visit and you're obviously pregnant. But that's not foolproof, it's not a systematic way to ensure screening for all pregnant women, and it may also not occur in time to prevent the worst effects of gum disease and its interactions with your pregnancy.

Why do I say it may not be in time? Because the current evidence shows that the presence of gum disease at 21 to 24 weeks into the pregnancy is associated with preterm delivery. By that point, it's a significant risk. Women with pre-existing periodontal disease in the second trimester increased their odds of prematurity from four and a half to seven times.[21]

There is even some later evidence suggesting that pregnant women who have gum disease between the 15th and the 20th weeks are already at high risk of premature birth. This has been confirmed by finding elevated levels of immune response markers for periodontal infection in the amniotic fluid.[22]

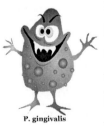

And, if you're of African American descent, it's even more important to get screened early, ideally even before you are pregnant. African Americans consistently have higher rates of preterm and low birth weight deliveries. Now, we have data showing that higher antibody levels against P. gingivalis in the midtrimester are associated with prematurity.[23]

P. gingivalis

Emphasizing the need for early detection, recent research has found that the more the gum disease progressed throughout the pregnancy, the more severe the outcome in terms of preterm delivery. In fact, the worse the gum disease gets, the more likely you are to have a very preterm birth[24], which is defined as delivery before the 32nd week of pregnancy.[25]

Similarly, the more of your mouth affected by periodontal disease, the greater the risk of delivery a premature baby. Women who have what's referred to as generalized periodontal disease, which means that it affects at least 30 percent of their mouth, have even higher risks of preterm delivery.[26]

Another factor that many women find frightening, and rightly so, is the discovery that oral infection organisms can be transferred to the fetus. Investigators have found that, in cases where a pregnant woman's immune response fails to engage and check the infection, the infection translocates into the fetus. They believe that this then becomes the primary cause of prematurity in these cases.[27]

Perhaps even scarier is the fact that, as toxins and other products generated by oral bacteria enter the bloodstream, they cross the placenta and harm the fetus. This is in addition to the mother's immune response cascade, which can also trigger preterm delivery.[28]

Gum disease can cause other pregnancy problems in addition to prematurity. Pregnant women who have severe periodontal disease, or whose periodontal disease progressed during their pregnancy, were at much higher risk – more than double, in fact – for preeclampsia.[29] This is a condition in which your blood pressure rises sharply, there's swelling in your face, hands and feet, and other effects may signal serious problems with the pregnancy. Untreated, it can turn into eclampsia, which can threaten the life of both the mother and the fetus.[30]

The Good News

There is a silver lining here. Periodontal therapy can safely be provided during pregnancy, and it works.

Treatment can be provided safely to improve the oral health of the mother and, by extension, reduce the risk of preterm delivery. The fact is that there is no evidence of a down side to treating gum disease during pregnancy.[31]

At the risk of sound crass, this is a no-brainer, a gimme and a two-fer all rolled into the single act of taking care of your teeth.

There are signs that this concept is catching on in the healthcare world. One relatively recent medical article informed physicians that there is compelling evidence pointing to dental therapy to control gum disease as a potential strategy to reduce preterm labor.[32] I believe we'll see even more of this as the evidence continues to mount and it gets more widely distributed throughout the healthcare professions.

In fact, recent research has found some of the strongest evidence so far. One study that provided periodontal treatment for pregnant women evaluated whether the treatment itself could interfere with the pregnancy term and the baby's weight. What they found was startling. There was no statistical difference at all between the healthy control group and the group of mothers who were treated for gum disease during pregnancy. What emerged as the smoking gun was in the group of pregnant women who had gum disease but weren't treated. Nearly 80 percent of them delivered a preterm low birth weight baby.[33]

Another study showed that women who were treated for gingivitis before their 28th week of pregnancy had a significantly lower incidence of premature birth. This is particularly important because gingivitis is the earliest form of gum disease. The study demonstrates that if an oral infection is diagnosed at any time during pregnancy, it should be treated as soon as possible.[34]

Even though this study focused on the 28th week mark, I suggest you get a full oral screening as soon as you decide to plan a pregnancy or, if you're already pregnant, as quickly as you can make an appointment with your dentist. Remember the earlier research we discussed that showed an association between gum disease at 15 weeks? It's never too soon to get it checked.

If you want a healthy baby one good way to start is with a healthy mouth.

Testimonials: Heather Pennington and William Boyd

Looking better and feeling better

Embarrassment gets lots of people into my office as does pain. And often they're intertwined – pain as a result of an injury that leaves your teeth looking less than perfect or pain as the result of long term dental neglect due to fear.

Heather Pennington was a patient who needed dental work because of an injury. **William Boyd** needed dental work because of neglect. But the one comment they both shared with me was embarrassment – both talked about how embarrassed they were by how their teeth looked.

Heather, a pre-teen when she chipped her two front teeth in a pool accident, told me how embarrassed she was to smile or talk after chipping her teeth. She'd been racing a friend to the other side of the pool without goggles, lifted her head to get a breath and hit the cement side of the pool. Brave girl that she is she didn't cry, but she sure was scared when she realized she'd chipped her teeth.

Here's her story in her own words. "I was kind of scared because I thought they would pluck my teeth out and put new ones in. They called my name and I followed the dentist into the long hallway to my room. I sat in a dental chair and first they had to clean around my teeth. After that they numbed my mouth and then it was down to work. They made sure that there were no cavities and then they put caps where my teeth were chipped.

"When it was all over I felt so relieved. It went great and the only thing that hurt even a little was when they numbed me, but it was great afterwards. I love my new teeth and the smooth feeling I now get when my tongue goes across them."

Heather's story is typical of people of any age who have teeth damaged in an accident. They've had a great smile and they want it back.

For people who neglect their teeth, the story's not all that different. When they smile they're embarrassed, but if they realized the toll their dental neglect can be taking on their physical health by avoiding dental care – they'd be scared. Usually they arrive at my office experiencing both physical pain and embarrassment about what I'm about to see.

William Boyd was one of those patients. He dreaded a dental visit so he just didn't go. Years and years of neglect took its toll and after a long painful weekend he ended up in my chair the next week.

At the point where he visited our office he was suffering from two types of discomfort – serious physical pain and serious embarrassment about the state of his mouth.

Five years later we'd been through a lot together. Bill's had numerous dental procedures including implants, gum surgery, cosmetic teeth replacement and a complete tooth restoration. It's been a long journey, but finally he's got a mouth and a smile he's proud of.

How does Bill describe his experiences? Here's what he says about the first visit to our office: "The fateful day arrived with the personal and physical discomfort each about equal in intensity. After a brief discussion and a look at the problem, Dr. Martin's first comment was 'let's get this taken care of right away,' and so it was. This was the beginning of what became known as 'The Journey' toward improved dental health and hygiene for me.

"What is so amazing about this story? On a scale of Good to Worse, with one being Good and ten being Worst, the condition of my gums and teeth would have been generously considered a ten. Despite this condition, Dr. Martin's focus was about how to help me, not how to embarrass me, lecture me or make me uncomfortable about the obvious. From that day forward and over the next five years we went through numerous procedures together that today make be look and feel better than I had ever imagined possible.

"Along the way Dr. Martin and his staff became like family. Would I do this again? Yes. Was it worth it? Yes. Would I recommend Dr. Martin and his staff? Absolutely.

"My advice to anyone who fears the dentist is to cast aside your thoughts about discomfort and take advantage of the changes and advances in dental care. Any journey begins with the first step and one that results in a perfect smile is a journey worth taking."

---

1 U.S. Department of Health and Human Services, Centers for Disease Control and Prevention, National Center for Health Statistics, Birthweight and Gestation, http://www.cdc.gov/nchs/fastats/birthwt.htm accessed 6/29/2008

2 Medline Plus, Premature Babies, http://www.nlm.nih.gov/medlineplus/prematurebabies.html#cat22, accessed 6/29/2008

3 March of Dimes, Learn the Facts – Complications in the Newborn, http://www.marchofdimes.com/prematurity/21191_6306.asp, accessed 6/29/2008

4 U.S. Department of Health and Human Services, Centers for Disease Control and Prevention, National Center for Health Statistics, Press release, Overall Infant Mortality Rate in U.S. Largely Unchanged, May 2, 2007, http://www.cdc.gov/nchs/pressroom/07newsreleases/infantmortality.htm, accessed 6/29/2008

5 Los Angeles Best Babies Collaborative, Healthy Births Initiative Blueprint, http://www.first5la.org/docs/Projects/HB/LABBCHealthyBirthsBluePrint.pdf

6 Ibid.

7 Ibid.

8 Ibid.

9 Gibbs RS, The relationship between infections and adverse pregnancy outcomes: an overview, Annals of Periodontology, December 2001, Vol. 6, No.1, Pages 153-163

10 Dasanayake AP, Boyd D, et al., The association between porphyromonas gingivalis-specific maternal serum IgG and low birth weight, Journal of Periodontology, 2001, Vol. 72, no. 11, pp. 1491-1497

11 Merriam-Webster Medical Dictionary, IgG, http://medical.merriam-webster.com/medical/igg, accessed 6/29/2008

12 Bogess KA, Is there a link between periodontal disease and preterm birth?, Contemporary OB-GYN, Aug.1, 2003

13 MedicineNet.com, Prostaglandin E2, http://www.medterms.com/script/main/art.asp?articlekey=24892, accessed 6/29/2008

14 Op. cit., Interleukin-1, http://www.medterms.com/script/main/art.asp?articlekey=11521, accessed 6/29/2008

15 Medline Plus, Intrauterine Growth Restriction, http://www.nlm.nih.gov/medlineplus/ency/article/001500.htm, accessed 6/29/2008

16 Offenbacher S, Lieff S, et al., Maternal periodontitis and prematurity, Part I: Obstetric outcome of prematurity and growth restriction, Annals of Periodontology, 2001, Dec;6(1):164-74

17 New York University (2009m, April 6) New Evidence Of Periodontal Disease Leading to Gestational Diabetes, Science Daily. Retrieved September 17, 2009, from http://www.sciencedialy.com/releases/2009/04/090404164115.htm.

18 Boggess KA, Edelstein BL, Oral health in women during preconception and pregnancy: Implications for birth outcomes and infant oral health, Maternal Child Health Journal, 2006, September; 10(suppl 7): 169-174

19 Ibid.

20 National Guideline Clearinghouse, Routine prenatal care, http://www.guidelines.gov/summary/summary.aspx?ss=15&doc_id=11532&nbr=5973, accessed 6/30/2008

21 Jeffcoat MK, Geurs NC, et al., Periodontal infection and preterm birth : Results of a prospective study, Journal of the American Dental Association 2001 ; 132 :875-880

22 Dortbudak O, Eberhardt R, Periodontitis, a marker of risk in pregnancy for preterm birth, Journal of Clinical Periodontology, Volume 32 Page 45 – January 2005

23 Dasanayake AP, Russell S, Preterm low birth weight and periodontal disease among African Americans, The Dental Clinics of North America, 2003, vol. 47, No. 1 pp. 115-17

24 Offenbacher S, Boggess KA, et al., Progressive periodontal disease and risk of very preterm delivery, Obstetrics & Gynecology 2006;107:29-36

25 Mathews TJ, Menacker F, MacDorman MF, Infant mortality statistics from the 2002 period: linked birth/infant death data set, National Vital Statistics Report 2004;53:1-29

26 Jeffcoat M, Research presented today provides further evidence on the importance of good oral health in pregnant women, Press release, May 2000, American Academy of Periodontology Specialty Conference on Periodontal Medicine, Washington, DC, May 7, 2000

27 Madianos RPN, Lieff S, et al., Maternal periodontitis and prematurity, part II: Maternal infection and fetal exposure, Obstetrical & Gynecological Survey, 58(7):438-439, July 2003

28 World Health Organization, Adverse pregnancy outcomes and periodontal disease, http://www.whocollab.od.mah.se/expl/systpreterm.html

29 Boggess KA, Lief S, et al., Maternal periodontal disease is associated with an increased risk for preeclampsia, Obstetrics & Gynecology 2003;101:227-231

30 MedicineNet.com, Preeclampsia, http://www.medterms.com/script/main/art.asp?articlekey=11892, accessed 6/30/2008

31 Bobetsis YA, Barros SP, et al., Exploring the relationship between periodontal disease and pregnancy complications, Journal of the American Dental Association, vol. 137, Oct. 2006 Supplement, pp. 7s-13s

32 Yeo BK, Lim LP, et al., Periodontal disease – the emergence of a risk for systemic conditions: preterm low birth weight, Annals of the Academy of Medicine, January 2005, Vol. 34 No. 1

33 Gazolla CM, Ribeiro A, et al., Evaluation of the incidence of preterm low birth weight in patients undergoing periodontal therapy, Journal of Periodontology, 2007, Vol. 78, No. 5, pages 842-848

34 American Academy of Periodontology, Periodontal therapy may reduce incidence of preterm births, Media Release, Nov. 2005

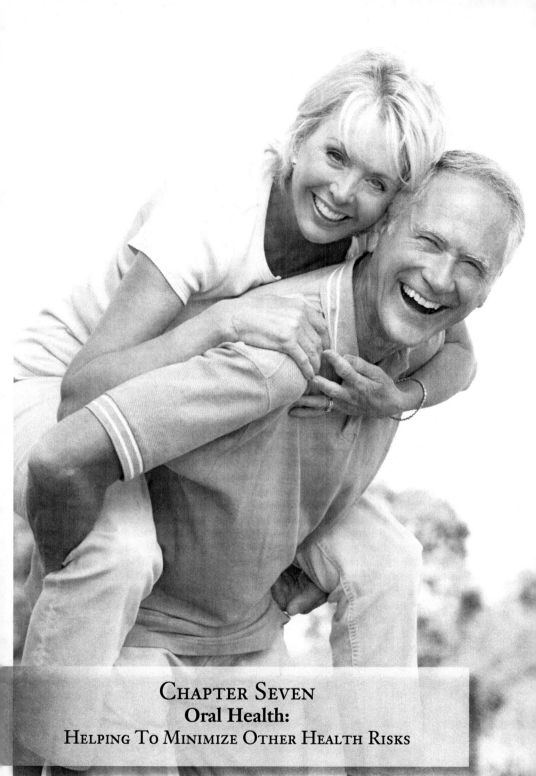

CHAPTER SEVEN
Oral Health:
HELPING TO MINIMIZE OTHER HEALTH RISKS

CHAPTER 7
Oral Health: Helping to Minimize Other Health Risks

Since 2006 there's been an increased focus on the links between periodontal inflammation and other diseases like diabetes, cancer, kidney disease, lung disease, obesity, osteoporosis, ulcers and arthritis.

Granted, there was a lot of research and focus on oral health and systemic disease links going on prior to 2006, some of which led to the first Surgeon General's Report on Oral Health in 2000 as well as a number of other reports of systemic disease links with oral health problems. But 2006 was a milestone year. It was then the American Dental Association and the American Medical Association held a joint conference to discuss the benefits of medicine and dentistry working together.

Not only does this kind of collaboration lead to better health for patients, it also has the potential to reduce the overall care of several chronic conditions. Various studies have linked obesity, kidney disease, lung disease, some cancers, osteoporosis, ulcers and arthritis to gum disease as well. Research continues to focus on the oral-systemic health connections, giving us all hope for improved understanding of just how dental care can help improve the overall care we and our physician colleagues provide you.

In this chapter we review current information on dental health and how it affects obesity, kidney disease, lung disease, cancer, osteoporosis, ulcers and arthritis. There is literally so much information available that it can be difficult to wade through, so I'll summarize the highlights in each area.

Obesity

Obesity and its increasing prevalence in the United States frequently make health headlines as a risk factor for a variety of diseases and the threat it poses to longevity.   It's a serious threat.

Today 60% of the United States population is overweight and about half of that group is heavy enough to be considered obese.

There is growing scientific evidence confirming the links between obesity and gum disease.

People whose bodies store their fat around the waist are more likely to have gum disease than other body types.

Inflammation response components that the body uses to fight disease, typically secreted by fat tissue, may be the key culprit in the interactions between gum disease, obesity and chronic health conditions.

While you often hear about obesity as a factor in heart disease, in some cancers, as a factor in high blood pressure and stroke and a myriad of other ailments, you don't often hear about it being linked to gum disease. But it's looking more and more like there is a connection.

In Europe, Dutch researchers have linked obesity to tooth decay, gum disease and dry mouth[1] and a German team of researchers did an extensive review of multiple studies that link obesity to gum disease. Their report[2], published in the Journal of Dental Research in 2007, cites research studies done as early as 1962 through 2005. The studies indicate various possible links between obesity and gum disease. Many of the laboratory studies these researchers cited have been supported by epidemiological studies of individuals living in Brazil, Japan and the United States.

The epidemiological study of United States residents determined that obesity could be a factor in periodontal disease and found a particularly strong association between obesity and gum disease in individuals between ages 18 and 34. In that same age group being underweight seemed to make subjects less likely to have gum disease.[3]

A recent study from the The Forsyth Institute[4] discovered new links between certain oral bacteria and obesity. This research looked at oral bacteria as a possible contributor to obesity. It demonstrated that the bacterial makeup of the saliva in overweight women differed from women who were not overweight. Researchers found one bacterial species, Selenomanas noxia, at levels over 1.05 percent in the overweight women. The researchers speculate that salivary bacterial changes may be indicators of developing an overweight condition and may, in fact, be a cause of obesity.

Whether obesity is a factor in gum disease or whether it may be caused by gum disease, much of what I've read suggests there's a correlation between where fat is stored in your body and gum disease. Individuals who carry extra weight around the waist – the classic apple shape – are more likely to experience gum disease than those who have a pear shaped body type.

Some researchers also believe there's a link between cytokines – the regulators of our body's response to disease and trauma – and gum disease. They theorize that proinflammatory cytokines – the kind that make disease worse – may play a key role in the relationship between gum disease, obesity and other chronic diseases. Those same proinflammatory cytokines are typically secreted by fat tissues.

Researchers continue to discover new cytokines and hormones that are secreted by fat tissue all the time, showing us how complex the body's endocrine system really is. Much of what we've learned over the past few years is that hormones and cytokines are involved in a variety of functions and diseases in the body and may be significant factors in the prevalence of obesity.

Chronic Kidney Disease

If you have missing teeth and if you have gum disease you are twice as likely to have chronic kidney disease as are your friends who don't have either of these problems.[5]

Who'd have thought that dental neglect was linked to chronic kidney disease? Lots of people are surprised by the connection. But it's significant as one of nine Americans suffers from chronic kidney disease, according to the National Kidney Foundation.

Most medical professionals see oral health problems as non-traditional risk factors for kidney disease, but a recent study by Dr. Monica Fisher and colleagues at Case Western Reserve University indicates gum disease is a predictor for chronic kidney disease.

The study was done with nearly 13,000 adults who had at least one risk factor for kidney disease. The theory behind the research was that the inflammatory response the body has to gum disease could mean that gum disease was a risk factor in developing chronic kidney disease.

Traditionally physicians have looked at other risk factors for kidney disease like diabetes, high blood pressure, overuse of pain killers, allergic reactions to antibiotics and drug abuse.

Among the participants in the study Dr. Fisher and colleagues developed, 3.6 percent had chronic kidney disease and six percent had gum disease. Over ten percent had missing teeth, 23.5 percent had high blood pressure and 36.4 percent were obese.

Those who had gum disease were nearly twice as likely to have chronic kidney disease (60%) and among those with missing teeth – another typical sign of dental neglect – some 85% had chronic kidney disease when compared with the research subjects without oral health risk factors.

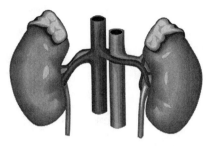

A Swedish study found that kidney disease patients had more dental problems than the study participants who did not have kidney disease. Moreover, their oral health issues developed before they progressed from the earliest stages of the disease to dialysis.

Other studies on kidney disease and gum disease suggest that caring for gum disease may be important in the treatment of kidney disease patients who have end stage renal disease and who are on dialysis.[6] These patients already high levels of inflammation in their system, which leads to heart problems and often heart disease related death. Reducing the inflammation these patients are experiencing by treating their gum disease may help physicians manage their overall treatment.

While more research is needed, this suggests just one more reason that keeping your mouth in good shape and taking care of your gums is key to a longer, happier, healthier life.

Lung Disease

If it's in your mouth it could be in your lungs. It's a very direct connection between the health of your mouth and the health of your body.

There's a lot of evidence that suggests that poor oral hygiene, the hundreds of species of bacteria that live and sometimes party in your mouth, and bacterial pneumonia may be linked. It's not surprising that bacteria growing in the mouth can be inhaled into the lungs to cause diseases like pneumonia. From there it's not a great leap to assume that neglect of your mouth and teeth and any oral health problem – like gum disease – could be connected to frequent bouts of respiratory disease. Many researchers believe that if your gums recede due to poor care of your mouth, you're a likely candidate for respiratory problems like pneumonia, emphysema and bronchitis.

Inhaling fine droplets from the mouth and the throat into the lungs is how most bacterial respiratory infections get started7. The germs in these droplets can breed and multiply within the lungs. This can cause miserable lung infections or, for people who already have some type of lung disease, it can make their problems worse.

If you have any type of lung disease, especially something like chronic obstructive pulmonary disease, what you're inhaling from your mouth into your lungs could cause you lots of misery or even threaten your life. The damage already done to your lungs by chronic obstructive pulmonary disease may have left you less able to eliminate bacteria from your lungs. This is serious stuff – especially if you or anyone in your family is vulnerable. Chronic obstructive pulmonary disease is the sixth leading cause of death in the United States.

Yet there is good news too. For people with normal lungs, it's possible that brushing and flossing your teeth can keep you from getting respiratory disease.

Given the evidence we already have on the connection between gum disease and lung disease, it's an area of oral and systemic health that is and will be studied as researchers continue to work on unraveling the oral health – physical health connection.

Cancer

Cancer is always a scary word. But it's possible that caring for your mouth, making sure you have good oral hygiene and treating any signs of gum disease could help you avoid developing cancer – including one of the deadliest – pancreatic cancer.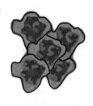

A study from the Harvard School of Public Health analyzed data from the Health Professionals Follow-up Study. This study has gathered health issue data from over 51,000 American men. Their findings, released in 2007, showed that men who had gum disease were 63 percent more likely to develop pancreatic cancer than those who did not have gum disease. Non-smokers who had gum disease were twice as likely to develop pancreatic cancer as those who did not have gum disease.

 Another study, released in May 2008, indicates that men with a history of gum disease had a 14% higher overall risk of cancer than those who didn't have gum disease whether they were smokers or non-smokers.

But there are other types of cancers that are related to gum disease as well. Recent research published in the British medical journal Lancet Oncology found that people who had gum disease also ran a 36 percent higher risk of lung cancer, even if they had never smoked. If they had fewer teeth than normal, indicating serious gum disease that resulted in tooth loss, their risk of lung cancer was 70 percent higher. The risk of kidney cancer was 40 percent greater. Risks for blood cancers – such as non-Hodgkin lymphoma, leukemia and multiple myeloma – were 50 percent higher.

Not surprisingly oral cancers are more likely to strike people with gum disease, according to a University at Buffalo study released in 2003. One of the study co-authors, Dr. Sarah Grossi, noted that previous research had shown associations between other infections and cancer such as H. pylori and stomach cancer, and the human papillomavirus and cervical cancer. While many people don't think oral cancers are too serious, they're much more deadly and much more widespread than many realize. Organizations who track cancer deaths report that one person dies of an oral cancer every hour of every day.

Now another study suggests gum disease may play a role in the risk of head and neck cancers. Researchers report that people diagnosed with head and neck cancers are much more likely to also have chronic periodontitis – even after taking into account cancer risk factors like smoking.

The connections that we're beginning to see between gum infections and the body-wide immune response they trigger, creating an inflammation response that can give off chemical signals that promote tumor growth, give me great hope that we can use good oral health practices and hygiene as one of the many tools in the battle against cancer.

Another issue for cancer patients are the side effects of treatment that affect your mouth and have the potential to interfere with your cancer treatment and affect you overall quality of life, whether it's the development of dry mouth or a life threatening infection.

While the battle against cancer will never be so simplified as just good oral hygiene, I look ahead to a day when it's acknowledged as an important weapon in the fight.

Osteoporosis

Researchers now think that osteoporosis, or loss of bone density, may be linked to bone loss in the jaw and that can lead to tooth loss because of the damage to the structure supporting the teeth.

Of course your teeth need a strong foundation. And we do know that gum disease by itself can weaken that foundation. Remember in Chapter Two where we talked about the structure of your mouth and how your teeth, bones and ligaments all work together?

We also talked about how gum disease can start to erode that structure. Here we have a different kind of erosion of the structure of your mouth. The studies that have been done suggest that the loss in bone density that signifies osteoporosis means a weaker foundation for the teeth. That can lead to tooth loss, and is considered one of the reasons one-third of all adults age 65 and older have lost teeth.

While the relationship to tooth loss and gum disease is well-documented, it's less clear how gum disease and skeletal bone density is linked. Researchers speculate that the loss of mineral density in the jaw bone leaves bone more susceptible to periodontal bacteria. That could increase the risk for gum disease and tooth loss. This is significant for women in a couple different ways. It's important for women who have osteoporosis because they are three times more likely to experience tooth loss than those who do not have osteoporosis. It's also a major concern for postmenopausal women with gum disease because the bacteria that's causing your gum disease can make you more likely to experience bone loss in the mouth. Without treatment that greatly increase the chances of tooth loss.[8]

Another concern is that we don't yet know if osteoporosis treatments have the same effect on bones in the mouth as they do on other bones.

And there is some concern about bisphosphonates, which are used to treat osteoporosis. They've been linked to the development of osteonecrosis of the jaw, although that's mostly shown up in people getting large doses of them for treatments such as cancer. It's rare for people taking oral bisphosphonates to treat osteoporosis to experience osteonecrosis of the jaw.

Lest you think gum disease and its effect on bones is an issue only for older women, it's not. It can be an issue for younger women who take oral contraceptives. A study of women age 20-35 found that those who used oral contraceptives had poorer periodontal health than women the same age who did not use oral contraceptives.9

HIV-1 Infection

Recent research by scientists at Nihon University in Tokyo suggests that gum disease, which is among the most prevalent microbial diseases in the world, may play a role as a risk factor for HIV-1. Their research suggests that gum disease can act as a risk factor for HIV-1's reactivation in people who have a latent HIV infection and may contribute to the development of AIDS.

Ulcers

The bacteria that cause stomach ulcers may also play a role in gum disease and vice versa. If you've got pockets in your gums it's likely that you've got Helicobacter pylori or H. pylori, the bacteria associated with stomach ulcers.

So it's not a big leap of faith to assume that if you've got a lot of bacteria in your mouth causing gum disease, those same bacteria may decide to take a little side trip and head for your stomach. When they do, they can play havoc and cause stomach ulcers or, if you've had ulcers before, cause them to return.

H. pylori infections increase with age and are also common in people who live at or near the poverty level.

Arthritis

Missing teeth, gum disease, jawbone loss and rheumatoid arthritis often are connected and some researchers think that a bacterial infection may trigger rheumatoid arthritis in some patients. This is not new thinking. Over 2,000 years ago Hippocrates suggested arthritis could be cured by removing infected teeth. Of course Hippocrates didn't have all the dental treatment tools that we have today. But given what we've learned about gum disease and arthritis, his theory certainly holds some weight.

Rheumatoid arthritis patients are twice as likely to have gum disease and some jawbone loss – from moderate to severe – compared with individuals who don't have rheumatoid arthritis.10 Researchers also found that rheumatoid arthritis patients averaged 11.6 missing teeth. That compares with an average of 6.7 missing teeth for individuals who don't have rheumatoid arthritis.

Some researchers believe the immune system and inflammation are key factors in both arthritis and gum disease. Meanwhile, no one is ready to say that periodontal disease causes rheumatoid arthritis, but I think most medical and dental professionals would agree that the relationship between bacterial infection in the mouth and arthritis is definitely worth further study.

It's long been a theory among dental professionals that people with arthritis may have poorer oral hygiene than people who do not have arthritis because it is more difficult for them to brush and floss as easily. Researchers are divided on this. In one study scientists found no significant differences in plaque accumulation between rheumatoid arthritis patients and the control group of individuals who did not have arthritis.[11] Another study found that oral hygiene could only partly account for the increased periodontal disease among rheumatoid arthritis patients.[12]

Recently researchers have found that treating severe gum disease may help rheumatoid arthritis suffers – alleviating some of the symptoms of both diseases. Scientists report that patients who were treated for their gum disease showed improvement in the severity of their arthritis and in their inflammation markers – no matter what medications the patients were also taking for arthritis relief.

There are other issues with arthritis that can make your oral health challenging. Patients with arthritis pain in the jaw joint can find that chewing firm foods is more difficult. As a result patients often eat softer, more calorie dense foods that can trigger weight gain and all its accompanying health issues. Plus, arthritis in your jaw can also make it more difficult to keep your mouth open for any type of extensive dental procedures.

If you've been diagnosed with arthritis, chances are you take high dosages of aspirin or other anti-inflammatory drugs. Or you may take antibiotics, steroids or other drugs. Anti-inflammatory drugs may cause severe bleeding after dental surgery. And antibiotics and steroids can weaken your immune system. Steroid therapy may make it harder for you to cope with a stress reaction, which some patients experience after dental procedures.

If you have arthritis be sure your dentist knows about your condition, how you're managing it and any drugs you take.

Sleep Apnea and Snoring

When Uncle Henry falls asleep on the living room sofa after Sunday dinner and snores so loudly that he drowns out the football game, it may not be just an occasion for grins and giggles around the family circle. It could actually signal a life-threatening condition. If you want Uncle Henry around for a few more years, you may want to encourage him to see his dentist or his physician about a condition called sleep apnea.

Known clinically in its most common form as obstructive sleep apnea, or OSA, it can be closely linked to periodontal disease. Good oral health care can be an important part of treating it before something serious happens to Uncle Henry.

As many as 18 million Americans are affected by sleep apnea, and an estimated 10 million haven't been diagnosed.[13] OSA can actually stop a person's breathing 30 or more times each hour during sleep, each

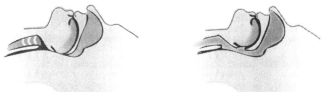

Sleep Apnea   Normal Airway

interruption typically lasting 10 to 20 seconds. In general, people who have OSA can't get enough air through their nose and mouth because of an obstruction. Their blood oxygen level can drop significantly. When they start breathing again, it's often accompanied by a snort or a choking sound.[14] Researchers have connected OSA with high blood pressure, heart attack and stroke.[12] In children, sleep apnea can contribute to attention deficit hyperactivity disorder.

Another health issue related to sleep apnea has major implications for our increasingly overweight population, and especially for those who have diabetes. Sleep apnea can be affected by a brain chemical called leptin. This hormone plays a crucial role in modulating appetite. It reduces the body's production of another chemical, a powerful appetite stimulator called neuropeptide Y. As leptin inhibits neuropeptide Y, your body tends to expend more energy and tends to increase metabolism of fat.[15]

But as your body accumulates more fat, it becomes resistant to the effects of leptin. And, as you gain weight, the excess body fat begins to affect your respiratory system in several ways and becomes a major risk factor for OSA. As OSA increases your fatigue level, you're less likely to be active and get the exercise you need to burn fat. Weight gain continues to pile up, and the whole cycle perpetuates itself and just gets worse.

One of the significant effects of OSA on dental health is the fact that many people who have sleep apnea tend to grind their teeth in their sleep more than those who don't have this condition. The medical term for this is sleep bruxism. If it occurs frequently enough and severely enough, it can cause jaw problems, tooth damage and headache. Because it happens during sleep, many people aren't even aware that it's going on so it can be tough to diagnose before they begin to experience complications.

Symptoms include worn, flattened or chipped teeth, increased sensitivity in your teeth, pain or tightness in your jaw muscles, earache caused by the severe jaw muscle contractions, chronic pain in your face and damage to the tissue on the inside of your cheek. If you have any of these signs, talk with your dentist right away. Don't be surprised if the diagnosis process starts pointing a finger towards sleep apnea.

One frequent treatment for OSA is a dental appliance that repositions the mandibular, your jaw. When you sleep, all your muscles relax. This includes your muscles in your airway. And, if you sleep on your back, these relaxed muscles can form an obstruction that restricts your breathing. By pushing the lower jaw forward, the appliance helps open the airway to allow more normal breathing.[16]

The mandibular appliance is the first line of defense against slight to moderate sleep apnea. It's likely to be the first thing your dentist will use to treat this condition. Unfortunately, periodontal problems – especially those severe enough to loosen a tooth – can keep you from using a dental appliance.[17] Even if you can use this appliance, it can change your bite over a long period of time and can also cause changes in your temperomandibular joint (TMJ).

Yet, alternative therapies can be more involved. One of the other typical treatments is called continuous positive airway pressure, or CPAP. A CPAP device requires you to wear a mask while you sleep. The mask is hooked to an air pump that gently blows air with enough pressure to keep your throat open.

The problems with CPAP are tw fold. First, compliance is terrible. Only about 30 percent use it consistently. The second issue is that it can cause TMJ pain because of the way the mask pushes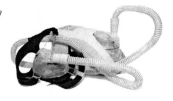

on the jaw. One type of CPAP mask fits only over your nose. It can push against your upper jaw with enough force that, over time, it can result in your front teeth actually tilting forward.

Used together, the dental appliance and CPAP are a more powerful combination. The appliance opens the airway enough that the pressure of the CPAP pump can be significantly reduced. Many may find it a more comfortable approach.

Other treatments for OSA can be invasive. Sometimes, surgery is recommended as a way to open your airway so you're less likely to have obstructions that stop your breathing.[14]

Another way periodontal disease plays into sleep apnea is associated with something called amyloidosis. This is a somewhat rare inflammatory disorder in which proteins called amyloids are abnormally deposited in various tissues. This buildup can cause serious changes.

Researchers have documented it as a cause of severe periodontal disease. The link with gum disease and sleep apnea involves the tongue. In amyloidosis, about 20 percent of people will develop an enlarged tongue. Not only can this interfere with speaking and swallowing. By posing an even larger airway obstruction during sleep, it can also cause sleep apnea.[18]

Your Mouth Is Integral to Your Body and Your Health

When we look at all the diseases that may be linked to gum disease and oral hygiene it's staggering. Many of the diseases that may be influenced by the quality of your oral health are some of the most serious we face as a society, including diabetes, heart disease, kidney disease, lung disease… the list goes on.

Not only are these diseases expensive to treat. They're also painful, often debilitating and can be fatal. Chronic disease saps strength and energy and limits enjoyment of life.

Throughout this book I've tried to guide you through some of the knowledge we have today on just how tightly oral health and physical health are linked. Today we have a much better understanding of how caring for your oral health also can help you in caring for your overall health.

As medical professionals we are learning daily about the results of new research. We're redefining the boundaries between oral health care and general health care.

What is clear is that your mouth is an integral part of your body – and your health. Pain and infection in your mouth can affect your entire body and may play a major role in other diseases. As dental care professionals we need to be opening dialogues with our colleagues throughout the medical field and creating team approaches that have only the patient's best welfare in mind.

Sharon Barkley Fosters' Story

Gum disease got the best of my teeth

There are lots of reasons people don't come to my office until it's a crisis. There's fear, embarrassment, cash shortages – I've heard all the reasons. Interestingly enough, reprimands are a big reason that people don't get to a dentist when they should.

That always bothers me – I know some of my fellow practitioners and their staff members lecture patients who come in with a neglected mouth. But that doesn't solve the problem. For whatever reason someone neglects their teeth, it's a reason that's mean-

ARE YOUR TEETH KILLING YOU

ingful to them. Our job as dental professionals is to help remove their concerns and get them on the path to a healthy mouth.

When Sharon Barkley Foster came to my office she definitely needed work. She came at the urging of family and friends. And I'm glad she did. Here's her story:

"I'd had orthodontia that required me to have some permanent teeth pulled. And I lost more teeth in a golf club accident. In total I lost eight teeth. I needed a bridge after the accident but I was already fearful of dentists.

"Of course my teeth shifted and eventually the neglect of my teeth led to gum disease. I began losing teeth one by one. I could only eat soft food and brushed gingerly in fear of losing another tooth. My once pretty smile was gone and I hid my mouth behind my hand when I spoke.

"After eight years of this my family and friends began urging me to see a dentist. Dr. Martin's approach, which was 'here's the problem and here's how we can resolve it' was just what I needed. No reprimands and no lectures.

"Because I'd let my mouth go so long, he had to extract my teeth, place implants in my lower jaw and attach a customized denture. It was expensive, but it was necessary.

"With my dental fears, I wasn't looking forward to the surgery, which took several hours. But it was amazingly painless. I had more discomfort from having my mouth open so long and so many hands in my mouth than I did from the extractions.

"So while I would have been a perfect patient to reprimand, and I'm a textbook example of how damaging gum disease can be to your entire mouth, today I have a great smile and a healthy mouth. But trust me, it would have been better and easier had I not neglected my mouth for so many years."

Sharon's story is one that often happens. Sometimes you can't save teeth that are too badly damaged. But there are lots of new dental techniques that help us restore our patient's mouth and give them a great smile, even when there isn't much to start with.

---

1 Oral aspects of obesity, International Dental Journal, Volume 57, Issue 4, 2007

2 Obesity, Inflammation and Periodontal Disease, Journal of Dental Research, 86(5) 400-409, 2007, http://jdr.iadrjournals.org/cgi/content/full/86/5/400, accessed 6/2/9/08

3 Obesity and Periodontal Disease in Young, Middle-Aged and Older Adults, Journal of Periodontology, May 2003, Volume 74, Number 5, Pages 610-615, http://www.joponline.org, accessed 6/29/08

4 Forsyth Institute (2009, July 9). Is Obesity An Oral Bacterial Disease? Science Daily. Retrieved September 17, 2009, from http://www.sciencedaily.com/releases/2009/07/090708153240.htm

5 Periodontal Disease and Other Nontraditional Risk Factors for CKD, American Journal of Kidney Diseases, Volume 51, Issue 1, pages 45-52, http://www.ajkd.org/article/S0272-6386(07)01368-6/abstract, accessed 6/29/08

6 Importance of periodontal disease in the kidney patient, New York University College of Dentistry, www.pubmed.gov, http://www.ncbi.nlm.nih.gov/pubmed/11803168?dopt=Abstract, accessed 6/29/08

7 Gum Disease and Respiratory Diseases, http://www.perio.org/consumer/mbc.respiratory.htm, accessed 6/29/08

8 Bacterial Species in Subgingival Plaque and Oral Bone Loss in Post Menopausal Women, Journal of Periodontology 2007, Volume 78, Number 6, Pages 1051-1061, http://www.joponline.org/doi/abs/10.1902/jop.2007.060436, accessed 6/30/08

9 Current Oral Contraceptive Status and Periodontitis in Young Adults, Journal of Periodontology 2007, Volume 78, Number 6, Pages 1031-1036, http://www.joponline.org/doi/abs/10.1902/jop.2007.060163, accessed 6/30/08

10 Relationship Between Rheumatoid Arthritis and Periodontitis, Journal of Periodontology, 2001, Volume 72, Number 6, Page 779-787, http://www.joponline.org/doi/abs/10.1902/jop.2001.72.6.779, accessed 6/30/08

11 Ibid.

12 Association Among Rheumatoid Arthritis, Oral Hygiene, and Periodontitis, Journal of Periodontology, June 2008, Volume 79, Number 6, Pages 979-986, http://www.joponline.org/doi/abs/10.1902/jop.2008.070501?prevSearch=keywordsfield%3A%28%22arthritis%22%29, accessed 6/30/08

13 American Association for Respiratory Care, Sleep Apnea Facts, http://www.yourlunghealth.org/lung_disease/sleep_apnea/facts/, accessed 7/2/08

14 Medline Plus, Sleep Apnea, http://www.nlm.nih.gov/medlineplus/sleepapnea.html#cat22, accessed 7/2/08

15 Marik PE, Leptin, Obesity and Obstructive Sleep Apnea, Chest, 2000;118:569-571

16 American Sleep Apnea Association, Treatment Options For Adults With Obstructive Sleep Apnea, http://www.sleepapnea.org/resources/pubs/treatment.html, accessed 7/2/08

17 Petit FX, Pepin JL, et al., Mandibular Advancement Devices : Rate of contraindications in 100 consecutive obstructive sleep apnea patients, American Journal of Respiratory and Critical Care Medicine, Vol. 166, pp. 274-278, (2002)

18 Khoury S, Dusek J, et al., Systemic amyloidosis manifesting as localized, severe periodontitis, Journal of the American Dental Association, Vol. 135, No. 5, 617-623, 2004

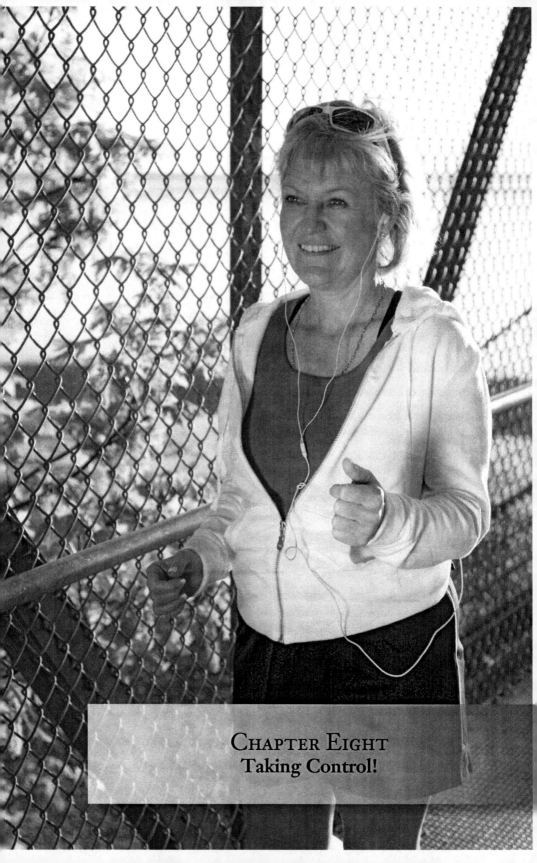

CHAPTER EIGHT
Taking Control!

CHAPTER 8
Taking Control!

When you take control of your physical health and your dental health, you're on your way to making sure you're doing everything you can to stay healthy.

Many times I have patients ask me how they can be sure they're getting the dental treatment they need. While some practitioners would be offended by that question, I'm glad to be asked because I know that a patient who asks me about their treatment is really concerned about staying healthy. It's a question that has only one good answer. You need a dentist who will pay special attention to your dental and health needs. If you don't feel that your dentist does pay special attention to the connection between your physical health and your dental health, it's time to have a discussion with him or her about your concerns.

If, as a result of that discussion, you still don't feel you're getting the kind of dental care you need it's time to start looking for a new dentist. After reading this book you'll have the knowledge you need to confidently start a conversation with your current dentist about your treatment or to interview new dentists. Meanwhile, in this chapter we'll discuss a few key points that you'll want to cover with whomever you chose as your dental care provider.

What Should You Look for In Your Dental Treatment?

Here are the things your dentist should do as part of your routine oral health care.

- Your dentist should show an interest in your general health and, at each visit, spend some time discussing the current state of your health and any changes in your health since your last visit. If your dentist hasn't asked you about your general health and doesn't spend at least a few minutes getting up to date during your repeat visits, you should initiate a discussion with him or her. Talk very directly to your dentist about any health concerns you may have and ask him or her if there are specific dental treatments that could help improve your health.

- Your dentist should adapt his or her diagnostic process when giving you your regular check ups to include baseline data about your health including any chronic problems like heart disease, cancer, kidney disease, ulcers and arthritis to name a few, and to evaluate how that's affecting your oral health. Your dentist should be considering all factors affecting your general health in your dental care. That's critical for your ongoing dental health and your physical health.

- Your dentist should be willing to talk with you about the oral health problems you have and whether your oral health could be linked to general health issues. For example: gum disease is more prevalent – and often more severe – in patients with chronic health issues like diabetes.

What Should You Do to Make Sure You Get the Dental Treatment You Need and Deserve?

- Find a dentist who is committed to staying up to date on the latest research results on the connection between oral health and physical health and between oral infection and inflammation and its overall effect on the body.

- Bring to your dental appointments the result of any tests from your physical that might be pertinent to your dental health such as your C-reactive protein blood tests results that measure the level of inflammation in your body.

- Encourage – insist on – open communications between your dentist and your physician. You may need to be the information conduit, bringing your medical records to your dental appointment and making sure you share with your physician what you learn at the dentist. But talk to both of these health care providers about your overall health, both dental and physical, and talk about how you can all communicate as a team. Keep your physician up to date about what you find out at the dentist and make sure your dentist is part of your health care team.

Inflammation: Its Affect on Your Oral and Physical Health

Inflammation is one of the hottest topics in medicine and dentistry today. That's not meant as a humorous comment either – inflammation is serious stuff. Research on inflammation abounds and we're learning more about it and its effect on the body almost daily. Moreover, we're now much more aware of the need to monitor and treat the symptoms of inflammation closely.

What does that have to do with oral health? Well gum disease is a source of inflammation that triggers the formation of the C-reactive proteins that I mentioned earlier. These proteins are the body's "first alert" system for fighting the onset of inflammation. The goal of your dentist and your physician should be to help you avoid inflammation bouts that can trigger a series of health problems.

When you monitor your health closely, do routine testing and encourage open, frank communications between your doctor, your dentist and yourself, you are more likely to find serious problems earlier, when they may be more treatable.

Your health care team should be monitoring your CRP levels regularly. It's especially important to keep close tabs on your CRP level after a periodontal treatment. Why? Because if your levels don't drop after treatment you may have other problems that need the attention of your primary care physician Certain cancers, including prostate, colon and pancreatic cancer, have all been found to be linked to elevated CRP levels. Now this sounds scary, but one of the scariest things about any of these cancers is when they go undetected until they are discovered at a point where they are almost untreatable.

Scientists continue to study C-reactive proteins. As a result, data from their research is released regularly, providing those of us in direct patient care with more and more information on just what this blood marker can tell us about our patients. That, as part of our diagnostic approach, helps us design continually improved treatments.

When your dentist and your physician work together, you will have a team working with you, helping you stay on track with your health care. If you have dental problems that require repeated visits to the dentist, working with your dentist and physician to establish a working team relationship can have real benefits as you'll be seeing your dentist often – maybe more than you see your physician. Your dentist can help you stay on track and also help keep your physician alerted to any changes in your health that may need medical attention. For your best health, the three of you need to be working together as a team.

What Else Should You Consider?

What dental treatments should you consider? One that I recommend for all patients – whether they're chronically ill or the proverbial picture of health – is a complete dental physical.   A complete dental physical may include:

- A clinical exam
- Multiple individual teeth x-rays, to give a complete look at the teeth and the area between them.
- A panorex x-ray to evaluate supporting bone structure in which the teeth roots rest, along with the sinus area
- Molds of your teeth are used to show the relationship of the jaw to the skull, tooth position and interferences to the chewing mechanism
- Registration of your bite mechanism
- Jaw joints health evaluation
- Oral cancer screening
- Decay evaluation
- Tests for clinching and grinding habits
- Periodontal (gum) disease analysis
- Bite mismatches
- A complete series of evaluation photographs
- Bite records for a mechanical jaw simulator for your bite
- A smile design analysis
- Tooth color, tooth size, shape, and contours evaluation
- Evaluation of smile to facial type, complexion and shape
- Evaluation of dental problems contributing to general overall body health

This may or may not be a necessary part of your dental evaluation. It really depends on the extent of your periodontal problems. But if you dentist suggests it, you'll want to consider it.

Going Beyond the General Checkup

Sometimes your dentist will suggest more extensive dental treatment after a complete dental physical. Most people don't volunteer for extra time in the dental chair, but if your dentist does suggest additional treatment, please take the time to discuss the treatment and how it may benefit you. Some of the names of the treatments for common dental problems like gum disease sound scary, so as part of your discussions with your dentist, ask him or her to tell you what the treatment actually entails and how it will help you. When you understand the benefits of such treatment, it makes it easier to consider having it done.

One effective treatment for gum disease is root planing and scaling, especially if your gum disease is not severe. What root planing and scaling involves is cleaning between the gums and teeth to the roots. It's usually done under local anesthetic and now it can be done with ultrasound rather than a scraping tool. Despite the scary name, planing and scaling causes little or no discomfort.

You may also want to talk to your dentist about the latest in new laser treatments that are being used in treating gum disease and reducing bacteria in the mouth. The use of lasers in the dental care arena is growing rapidly and new studies on the effectiveness of a variety of laser treatments for gum disease are being released frequently. Your dentist will have information on the most up to date treatments available.

Teaming Up for Health

Taking care of your oral health is as important as taking care of your physical health because the two are closely linked. Hopefully after reading this book you have a better idea of what to expect when you visit the dentist, what to ask your dentist about and the importance of getting your doctor and your dentist to work together as a team.

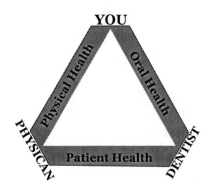

Think of an equilateral triangle. At each point is an important member of your diabetes health team. At the top of the triangle is you, the patient, because it's your health that we're concerned with. Your dentist and your physician are the other points in the triangle and you're all connected because the connection between your oral health and your physical health is so closely linked.

We've talked about what you as the patient should expect from your dentist. Now we'll talk about what you should do in your effort to improve both your oral and physical health and what you should expect of your physician in working with you and your dentist as part of your health care team.

Just as you did with your dentist, you need to initiate a conversation with your doctor about your concerns about your oral health and how that may be affecting your overall health.   Your doctor needs to know that you want to work with him or her and with your dentist to develop an integrated plan for staying healthy.

What to Discuss with Your Physician

Frankly, some physicians may balk at first when you ask them to be part of a health team with you and your dentist. Most of us in the medical and dental professions take a lot of pride in our work and can be a bit possessive about our patients. As a result, some care providers may initially resist the idea of forming a health care team, but these teams ultimately benefit you in your care and in managing your health.

Assure your physician that you're satisfied with the care you're getting (that is if you are satisfied) but that you want to see if a team approach that combines oral health and physical health treatments can improve your health or just help you stay healthier. Your doctor's first concern is your well being. Most are very willing to do what they can to try to help patients improve their health, especially if you have a chronic disease or a family medical history that could make you a likely candidate for chronic disease.

There are also some basic things you can as your doctor to do as part of your regular physical. One thing your doctor should do is screen for dental problems during your regular visits. These can be a series of simple survey questions and a quick look in your mouth for signs of inflammation and infection with your teeth. If your physician doesn't do an oral screening, ask for one. Doubling up on your health screenings is always a good idea and an oral screening is something many physicians now include with a regular check up.

Another thing to ask your doctor to do is to share the lab test results from your annual physical with your dentist and provide you copies for yourself. Your lab tests are not just your doctor's business. They're important markers of what's happening in your body. You need to know just what your lab tests show and have that interpreted by your doctor if all the acronyms and numbers are confusing. Plus you need to know what those numbers mean to your health.

What You Should Do

Remember that triangle we talked about that represents your health care team. You are at the top of the triangle and your doctor and dentist are at the other points of the triangle. You're all linked by the concern for your health.

That's why it's up to you to start the process toward better dental and physical health with a coordinated health approach between your dentist and your physician. You're critical to your health care team effort.

Let's face it, healthy behaviors often don't seem as interesting, fun or easy as unhealthy behaviors. After a tough day the couch is more appealing that a brisk walk. And when you're heading home tired a cruise through the drive in window of a fast food restaurant may seem appealing. But it's ultimately up to you to take responsibility for your health, both by living a healthy life style and by being your own personal advocate with your health care practitioners. You are the only one who knows how you feel and you need to communicate that to your team.

Take Control of Your Health – Your Key to Better Living

- Insist on cooperation between your health care providers. It's up to you to be your best health advocate. You're now ready to start that process with a series of questions and points that you'll want to discuss with your dentist and your doctor. During those discussions you'll ask practitioners to work together to integrate the care that you're given and to cooperate as a team in monitoring your health. As a patient you should insist on the cooperation of your health practitioners.

- Get active in your personal care. There's activism and there's activity. We've talked a lot about the activism: talking with your dentist your physician about your health and your desire to have a care team approach that includes your doctor, your dentist, and you. Now here's the tough part – the part that only you can do. You must be willing and able to take charge of your health to achieve your overall health goals. The first step in taking charge of your health is with healthy eating. What are your eating habits? Are you an activist for better food at your table? Have you talked with your doctor about healthy eating and what that really means?

You Are What You Eat

Checking with professionals about diet and exercise is important. If you just read news reports on nutrition you'd probably shift your diet weekly and be forever chasing the latest exercise fad. It seems like everyday there's something new being touted – what wasn't good for us last week is good for us today and vice versa.

There are some basic principles to making healthy food choices that won't just benefit you, but will also benefit your entire family.

- Put a lot of color on your plate with vegetables and fruits. Focus on non-starch vegetables like carrots, green beans, broccoli and spinach.
- Eat lean meats. Remove chicken and turkey skin and choose pork and beef cuts that end in "loin." They contain less fat than other cuts.

- Select non-fat dairy products like skim milk, non-fat cheeses and non-fat yogurt.
- Whole grain foods like brown rice and whole wheat pastas are better choices than their processed alternatives. Dried beans and lentils are great additions to your meals as well.
- Eat fish at least 2-3 times a week.
- Drink lots of water and if you drink sodas, make sure it's diet soda. Avoid sugary fruit drinks, sodas and teas.
- Cook with liquid oils, not solid fats. Solid fats are often high in saturated and trans fats. No matter what kind of oil you use, remember it's high in calories so monitor portions of foods with added fats. If you don't know how to determine how much fat is in your diet, ask for help in monitoring your fat intake.
- Limit desserts, full-fat ice creams and high calorie snack foods. Keep alternatives on hand and ready to eat (wash those baby carrots and trim that celery so you can just reach in the fridge and grab a handful).
- Learn about portion control and what actually constitutes one serving of a food. You can gain weight off healthy foods if you eat too much of them. Know what your calorie limits are. Your doctor or dietitian can help you determine the calorie levels and portion sizes you can eat.
- Talk with your doctor about working small, occasional treats into your diet.

The Next Step... Into the Exercise Zone

How's your activity level? What kinds of exercise do you do each day? No, walking from the car to the house doesn't count.

Any physical activity that gets you moving and active can qualify as exercise. That could be walking, dancing or working in your yard. You don't have to get an expensive gym membership, join a sports team or buy fancy equipment. You just need to get started. People who exercise report that they feel better, are stronger and have the endurance they need to get through the day. Plus exercise and the feeling of being fit offers you a mental boost as well.

Exercise is also credited with lowering blood pressure and cholesterol, which can reduce your risk for stroke or heart disease. And, people who exercise have stronger hearts, muscles and bones. Plus, it's a great stress reliever and absolutely necessary if you want to lose weight.

Best of all, it's never too late to get active. If you're not exercising right now, this is definitely something you should consider. Check with your doctor before starting any exercise program and then get going. Walking is probably the best, cheapest, easiest way to get started on an exercise regimen. Regular walking will:

- Increase your energy
- Help you relax
- Help reduce stress
- Improve your sleep
- Tone your muscles
- Help control your appetite
- Increase your calorie use
- Help prevent diabetes if you have been told you have prediabetes

While it's tough for most of us to find time to exercise, all you need is 30 minutes or so three times a week to get benefits from an exercise regimen. If you can exercise five times a week, that's even better. The key word is schedule: just like a lunch date or a meeting, exercise needs to go into your day planner. And while you may occasionally miss a day, it's important to get right back at it the next day until you've built such a good habit that exercise is as natural a part of your routine as going to bed at night and getting up in the morning.

To get going start with 15 minute walks. Stretch before you head out and build up your walking routine over time. For your first 15 minute walk, start with five minutes of slowly building up speed, five minutes brisk walking and five minutes "cooling down" as you slow back to your starting speed. Increase your walk time three minutes a week and use the added time each week to extend the "speed" segment of your walk. Finding an exercise buddy may help keep you motivated and get you out and going, especially on those days when you'd prefer to spend that extra half hour in bed or on the couch in front of the TV.

Lifestyle changes are difficult. Just about everyone has days when they don't eat like they should or get the exercise they need. So if you miss a day of exercise or have a forbidden food don't use that as an excuse to not eat healthily the rest of that day or the next day, or to get back on your exercise schedule the following day.

When you focus on positive results in your life you can improve your heart health, your dental health, and it just generally makes you feel better.

The Benefits of Healthy Living

Beginning investors are often told to keep close tabs on their investments because "Nobody cares about your money as much as you do."

Well, nobody should care more about your health than you. And frankly, the best care team in the world won't function without your active involvement and leadership.

You now have the information you need to talk with your dentist and with your doctor as well as some basic information on eating well and exercising for a healthier life.

The Key Is In Your Hands

The key to better living: to feeling better, to enjoying better health and a longer life is in your hands. It's a combination of efforts but the first steps are yours: eating healthy foods, exercising, begin being your own best medical advocate.

There's no better time to start than right now, and no better way to start than by initiating a conversation with your doctor and with your dentist at your next appointment. If you don't have an appointment scheduled soon, you may want to call and schedule a special consultation. Good health and a great smile are well worth it!

Testimonial: Bea Parrish

Rebuilding a beautiful smile.

When Bea Parrish came to our offices she knew a bit about us. Her sister had been a patient and had several implants done at our office. Bea was impressed with her success and came to have me take a look at her teeth.

"My sister thought Dr. Martin should look at me because I had lost a bridge. So I came in with her and soon I was also getting implants.

"My treatment and procedures by Dr. Martin include three implants. That was about 10 years ago. They have been absolutely wonderful, not the first minute of trouble with them."

Bea has had a lot of work done on her mouth, including six crowns across the front. She says "As to how I look, I think my six new crowns across the front are absolutely beautiful.

"I would say the process of the six new crowns was a little more than the three implants because I had been sick a lot the winter that I had them done. And, I am 10-12 years older than I was when I got the implants. However, Dr. Martin makes you feel very comfortable no matter how difficult the procedure.

"That's why I recommend his practice whenever people say they need a dentist. In fact, I give them directions to his office."

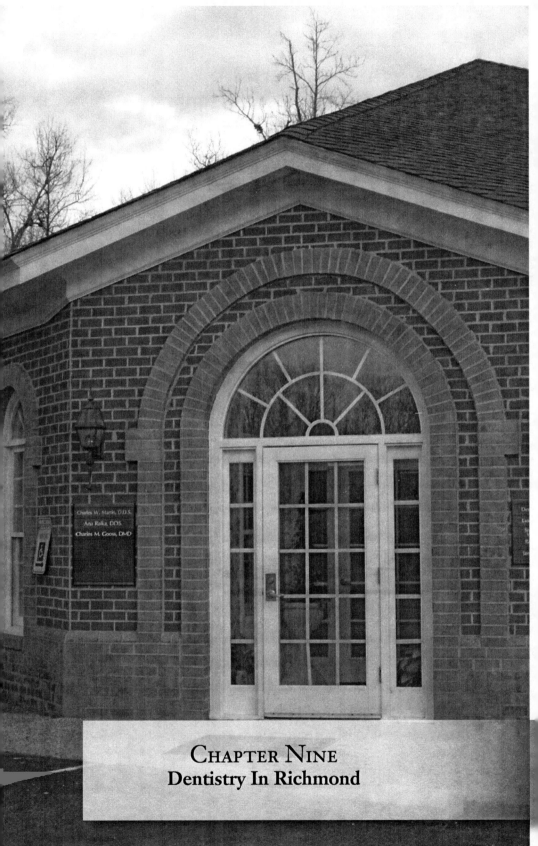

CHAPTER NINE
Dentistry In Richmond

CHAPTER 9
Dentistry In Richmond
by Dr. Charles Martin

L ong before I was a dentist, I grew and lost my baby teeth in a town called Bristol in southwest Virginia that borders Tennessee.

It was, and still is racing country. I can still remember being a kid and hearing the race cars thundering five miles down the road. We lived in an area where there were lots of small mountains. We were in a valley that went all the way down to the race track. We could hear the NASCAR races from my house.

I had a relatively uneventful childhood. I played football in elementary school. I didn't have a clue what I was doing, which is ironic since I became a college football player later on. But I didn't know the difference between a lineman and a back.

I read ravenously (and still do). I would buy Hardy Boys books and read one after the other in the series. I would just get a new one and sit down and read until it was done.

In those early years, my dentist was Dr. Poindexter. I remember him as a kind man, although he didn't talk a lot. His humble little office was at his home with one treatment room and a little waiting area all walled off from the rest of his house.

I remember noticing all his dental gizmos. And I remember getting my fillings placed and hearing the whirring of the drill and the smell it made. And there was a spittoon where you spit your rinse out. Aptly, Dr. Poindexter wore those glasses that had little magnifiers on them and I used to watch him work in the reflection they made.

Of course, back then, he used the silver amalgam material, which at that point was the best they could do. Thank God we have better stuff today. As I said, Dr. Poindexter didn't say a lot. His favorite saying was "Open." And he said it in a certain way. And "All right, you're done."

Academically, in high school, I was pretty good. In fact, that was when I first ran across my problem of being a jock versus being a student. And I didn't see why there should be a difference. I was just playing sports.

I ended up being lightly recruited to play college football. I say lightly because only a few colleges that were interested. So I went on a few recruiting trips. And I ended up playing at Virginia Tech.

When I did get to Virginia Tech, I didn't really know what to major in. I thought about Urban Planning. I thought about all sorts of things.

And then I remembered my dentist from high school, Dr. Hatcher. Ed Hatcher was a bit of a renaissance man. I got to know him pretty well because I dated his oldest daughter for about a year when I was in high school.

I admired him. I liked who he was and what he stood for. He was one of my dental heroes that really influenced me to change my major to biology.

When I first applied to dental school from college, they rejected me. But I wrote back and said, "No, you don't. And here's why you shouldn't."

I guess they weren't accustomed to that kind of thing, because I later got an interview and got into school that very same year they had sent me a rejection letter. I still have that letter. I guess that's one of my lessons I learned early in life was the power of persistence.

And that Dr. Hatcher, that I had admired, was certainly on my list of cheerleaders, because he ended up co-signing on a loan for me to go to dental school the first semester. It was for $8,500. Of course, that's long sense been paid back after I've been in practice now since 1979.

Dental school was interesting. And rigorous. My first semester there we had 36 semester hours in the first semester. Then it was followed by 52 semester hours. It was very much like being in medical school. We had gross anatomy, physiology, genetics, and biochemistry, all of it.

In the third year, we really started looking about the mouth, oral cavity and started to do surgery and work on teeth.

But early on I realized that dental school wasn't going to be enough. I knew I wanted continuing training. When you graduate from dental school you're only barely ready for a dental career. They've given you the basics. Most people probably think, "Well, you've graduated from dental school. You must be competent as a dentist."

In reality, your competence is something that must be built. So continuing training is vital.

So all along I emphasized studying different aspects of dentistry: medicine, behaviorism, physiology, the art of dentistry, the biomechanics and bio-physiology of it, how the bites and the jaw joints work.

All of this varied learning is an attempt to be a better professional, one who can see dental health in the context of people's lives. I've written other books. One, *Don't Sugar Coat It*, explains the connection between diabetes and dentistry, which is immensely important to understand, because diabetes makes dental health worse and poor dental health makes diabetes worse. Most people don't realize this.

And a second book, *This Won't Hurt a Bit*, which was written particularly to help educate consumers, particularly boomers, about how important their teeth are to them, their longevity, their quality of life and the quality of years in their life. And, of course, this book, all about the oral systemic connection, or how your mouth affects the rest of your health.

I also train other dentists. I'm a coach and consultant.

In 2007 I founded a national organization called Dentistry-ForDiabetics®, where we teach dentists all aspects of caring for the diabetic patient, especially those who have unanswered needs. And there are quite a few of them.

I'm also presently a columnist on dLife, which is a major diabetes portal online, where I explain what people need to know about their diabetes and their dental health.

Since I've been in private practice, I've also been a part time instructor at Georgetown University of Dental School and also at Virginia Commonwealth University School of Dentistry.

My present emphasis is on the patient needing major care: cosmetic dentistry, smile design, dental implants, and whole physiology of the chewing mechanisms. Most people don't realize how important all of this is.

To put it plainly, I'm the guy to come to when you have big problems. People that come to me are frustrated with their prior dental care, or when they've had failed treatment, have gum disease they can't get fixed, or are missing teeth or decay that won't go away.

ARE YOUR TEETH KILLING YOU

Unfortunately, most people know less about their teeth than virtually any other part of health care. Which is a real problem, because the mouth isn't just connected to the body, in many ways its health dictates the bodies health. Even medical schools don't teach that. And that's something I'm trying to change. It's why I wrote *Are Your Teeth Killing You?*

Amongst my designations I have a Master in the Academy of General Dentistry, a Diplomat of the International Congress of Oral Implantologists and a Fellow of the International Academy of Dental Facial Aesthetics.

I'm definitely a training and education junkie. My wife once told me, "Look, you've got so many plaques and certificates, it's costing us too much to frame them all." So, I don't even have them all up on my walls in my office.

I also put an emphasis on the behavioral and humanistic side of care so I can better understand people. So, I've studied the different personality assessments, including the Meyers-Briggs, the Predictive Index, and Neuro-Linguistic Programming. I even developed a philosophy about what a patient's experience should be. In fact, I'm one of the few dentists certified as an Experience Economy Expert, by the world famous Pine and Gilmore.

I've tried to learn from the best, from the people that have helped lead dentistry from the dark ages into the modern dentistry of today. Dr. L.D. Pankey probably is way up there in that pantheon. He was as much a philosopher and teacher of the <u>art</u> of dentistry as the science. And I've certainly worked to follow his principles throughout my career.

I've learned from Dr. Peter Dawson, who is a fine clinician and human being, who has been teaching fine dentistry and the how-to's and why's for a long time.

And I greatly respect Dr. Gordon Christiansen, a contemporary dentist who's worked in all facets of dentistry, tirelessly striving to improve the delivery and the care of the profession.

I've trained extensively with Dr. Carl Misch on dental implantology, since 1983. He's written the most popular, most often purchased textbooks in dentistry across the world, for his influence and affecting and impacting dentists and millions of patients from his work with teaching dental implants and how successful they can be. That's a major part of my practice now and has been for 25 years.

Dr. Omer Reed has helped many dentists like myself understand the importance of studying human behavior and how to communicate why people should care for their teeth. Because the reality is, no matter how good you are as a dentist technically, if you cannot communicate effectively or if you cannot help people understand what you're providing and why they should want it, you're sunk.

I chose to be a dentist for a many reasons. While I do enjoy working with my hands, and have a talent for working with them, the main reason I chose dentistry was to help people in a meaningful way. I wanted to make a difference. And that happens on a daily basis.

People often say, "You're a bit passionate about your job, don't you think?"

And I say, "Oh yes I am. I'm very passionate about doing it well."

I love modern dentistry because of the transformations we can effect. The transformations we make change a person's physical appearance. We change the way they think and feel about dentistry.

And that's vital, because your dental health affects every other part of their life. Smiles are a vital part of who you are and how you express yourself. And we help put smiles on people's faces. Not just physically on their face but a smile inside, in their heart.

We know that those transformations physically help our patients on an intellectual, emotional and spiritual level. I love helping people live better lives. I love the relationships and friendships I've built working with patients and other dentists that I coach and teach.

But there are some things about dentistry I'm unhappy with.

For one, I dislike the gap in understanding that the general population has about teeth and their health. The idea, "It's just a tooth," is sad and frightening. If it were just a finger or just a toe, I think people might have different thinking. It isn't just a tooth. It's a part of you, it's part of your health and part of who you are.

I also dislike when patients make me the target because of their previous dental history. Although fear rooted in past experience is understandable, people simply wouldn't do this with anyone else. Why, I can't say. I just know that dentistry is an emotional subject, and something many people are fearful of. So I bemoan the fact that bad experiences sometimes get in the way of our ability to take care of people.

In fact, one of the reasons I train other dentists is to help them create experiences for their patients that help erase those fears.

So what would I change about dentistry?

Chiefly, I'd like to change the fact that dentistry is misunderstood.

I'd like my books and my speaking to become a catalyst for change, a change for the better; more pleasure, more happiness, more understanding and frankly, a better life for my patients and the people I touch.

I know that the work that I do will have long lasting effects. We all want to make a difference and we all want to matter. So I love the fact that what I do as a dentist helps people laugh and love and experience life and all the richness it can hold.

Much has changed about medicine in dentistry. One of the biggest changes is that now we're understanding the connections between the mouth and the rest of the body - what we call the oral systemic connections.

The research is plentiful and we see it in our practices empirically. We see what occurs when other health conditions are present. And many times we're able to recognize problems in the mouth before anyone else sees them. So, we're actually able to detect early what's going on, even to the point now where there are some proteins in the saliva used to predict future cancers. It's very exciting.

It's an exciting time for dentistry, because we're now able to create beautiful smiles and beautiful teeth like we never had before because of new technology. We're able to replace missing teeth and even missing bone.

Another exciting thing is research in genetics and genomics which is leading us toward the ability to grow our own replacement organs and even teeth at some point.

We're also studying longevity, cellular aging, and what biology might tell us about cancer cells. And some scientists are now using the pulps inside of teeth – the nerves, blood vessels and connective tissue - to derive stem cells. I think that's very exciting.

So, the changes are incredible. It's really not the same profession it was when I went into it. It's better. And it's better on multiple levels, with our techniques, our technology, our understanding of human beings.

In many ways, patients don't have to put up with their problems or their old-school solutions like dentures.

Likewise, we can see in ways we never used to be able to see. In fact, in my own office I have a 3-D x-ray called the Cat Scan. And it's designed specifically for dental offices. With it we're able to evaluate and see in ways we never could before inside the mouth.

So, that's very exciting for us. And the new technologies keep coming, enabling us to perform better dentistry that lasts longer, looks better, and feels better.

I've had patients ask, "Well how long is this going to last?" And I will give an estimate, usually based on percentages. For example, "How long is my crown going to last?"

"Well, I can tell you that 92% of them are going to be there after 10 years."

"Well, that's a pretty good statistic."

Not many other areas of health care can make that kind of long-term claim. And we keep getting better - those percentages are improving.

What will dentistry be like in 20 years?

For one, I think we're going to find prevention will be even more important, not only to the mouth but to total body health. And I think that we're going to be able to detect problems earlier, which will help with both oral conditions and full systemic health.

We now know that the chronic low grade infections that a person has in his mouth causes inflammation that affects a person on multiple levels; cardiovascular, joints, upper respiratory problems, kidneys, etc. Virtually every part of the body is affected by the inflammatory pathway caused by chronic low grade infections you can't even feel. And these are common in the mouth.

Red flag: If your gums bleed when you brush, you've got a problem. Would you expect your scalp to bleed when you combed or brushed your hair? The answer's no. Your gums shouldn't either.

So, in the next 20 years, I think we're going to be able to provide longer lasting treatment to fix problems. I think it's going to be quicker, last longer, it's going to become easier and more comfortable to accomplish.

Because of the progress modern dentistry has made, we can help patients with major dental problems get their mouths back together again. We can eliminate infection, rebuild function and build smiles so they can feel good about whom they are.

Our offices here in Richmond were designed for comfort, with the goal to be opposite of what you expect with most dental offices. It has an Internet café, a patient theater, and a lounge. It looks different, smells different, and sounds different than old-fashioned dental offices.

We treat extremely challenging cases on a regular basis. When people ask, "Can anybody help me? Is there any hope for me?" We usually say yes.

And if there's only one thing I can say in words to people about dentistry, what would it be?

I'd like to say this. The past is the past. When you come to us as a patient, we won't be doing finger wagging or making belittling statements or making a person feel small. Those things are behind us. It's now time to start anew.

Old fashioned dentistry is basically dead. Long live the new day of comfort, health and beautiful smiles. We help people make intelligent decisions about their dental health and to have dentistry work for them instead of against them.

We turn frowning faces to smiling faces. And we increase the quality of life in the years and the years in the life. That's what we're particularly proud of; the beautiful smiles we make, helping the people keep their teeth for a lifetime, teeth that look good, feel good, that chew well and give you a peace of mind.

So, we can help you so you can have the beautiful smile and healthy teeth for life that you've always wanted.

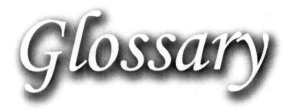

Glossary

A1C level The volume of glycated hemoglobin in your blood, used to measure the long-term average of blood glucose. Glycated red blood cells cause microvascular damage that can result in blindness, kidney disease, nerve damage, heart attack and stroke.

A1C variant A variation of A1C hemoglobin in the blood of people who are of African, Mediterranean or Southeast Asian heritage. This variation may cause false readings, either low or high. Medical professionals can take special steps to assure accurate results.

Alveolar bone The socket that your tooth sits in. It's actually two bones – one is the socket itself and the other is a structural support, sort of like the joists that sit on beams to provide support for the floor in your house. This structure provides a firm anchor point for your tooth.

Angiotensin A substance released by the outer surface of the kidney in response to microvascular damage caused by glycation. Angiotensin-converting enzyme transforms antiotensin into a powerful blood vessel constrictor that can cause high blood pressure.

Angiotensin-converting enzyme (ACE) inhibitors A class of drugs that prevent enzymes from converting angiotensin into its powerful vascular constrictor form, in order to prevent or reduce high blood pressure.

Angiotensin receptor blocker (ARB) A medication that reduces blood pressure by preventing converted angiotensin from constricting blood vessels. Often used if a person is not able to tolerate ACE inhibitors.

Antioxidants Nutrients that fight free radicals, oxygen-related byproducts of normal metabolism that can damage surrounding molecules, causing inflammation. Periodontal therapy now frequently includes antioxidants to keep free radicals in check and reduce inflammation.

Atherogenesis The process of forming plaques on the inner lining of the arteries. As the plaques pile up and spread across the arterial walls, they irritate the lining and cause inflammation. It triggers the body's inflammatory response and the cascade of adverse health events that go along with it.

Cementum The outer layer on the roots of your teeth. It's a fairly thin layer, a sort of dull pale yellow, and it has two main jobs – to protect the root of the tooth, and to provide a solid surface to attach to the tissue that holds your tooth in place.

Claudication Pain caused by lack of nutrients in muscle cells of the leg and foot, a result of microvascular damage by glycated hemoglobin cells. Progressive blockages can lead to tissue death and amputation.

Collagen One of the most common proteins in the human body, it is used to repair injuries to connective tissues such as periodontal ligaments. This element of the body's healing capacity is reduced in diabetics.

C-reactive protein (CRP) When the body senses inflammation somewhere in the system, it signals the liver to produce CRP. As inflammation worsens, the level of CRP in your blood rises. CRP is associated with both diabetes and gum disease, and is a predictor of heart disease and stroke.

Creatinine clearance A practical test to measure kidney function, this method monitors the level of a substance produced by the body that is filtered by the kidneys. When kidneys are damaged by microvascular effects of glycation, they are less able to filter creatinine which then remains in the blood at higher levels. This signals potential kidney disease.

Cytokines Proteins that the body uses to interact or communicate between different types of cells. Gum disease triggers proinflammatory cytokines. Diabetes triggers hyperinflammatory cytokines. These two cytokines interact to increase insulin resistance and make it more difficult for diabetics to control their blood glucose levels.

Diabetic retinopathy A frequent complication of diabetes that affects the retina. It is a microvascular effect involving glycated blood cells which can damage small vessels in the eye. Unchecked, it can lead to blindness.

End-stage renal disease A microvascular effect of glycation which leads to a gradual decrease in kidney function and, ultimately, kidney failure.

Gingivitis A mild form of gum disease. You may hear dental health professionals refer to the 'gingiva'. That's the clinical term for your gums. Gingivitis often develops when plaque builds up on your teeth at the gumline and irritates the gum.

Glomerular filtration rate Measure used to examine kidney function. Glomerules are tiny structures in the kidney which concentrate wastes from the bloodstream into urine. These structures are readily damaged by microvascular effects of glycation. Usually monitored in clinical practice through another measurement called creatinine clearance.

Glycation A byproduct of high blood sugar, in which excess glucose actually binds to the outside wall of cells in the bloodstream. Glycated hemoglobin blood cells are responsible for microvascular damage that can result in blindness and kidney failure.

Hyperglycemia High blood glucose, often referred to as high blood sugar.

Hypoglycemia Low blood glucose, the opposite of hyperglycemia.

Immune response The body's mechanisms and processes for fighting infection, including periodontal pathogens.

Immunoglobulins A class of antibodies employed by the immune response system.

Inflammation response Sensing irritation, the body responds with an automatic system that's a defense mechanism against inflammation. This is a complex set of events that send several different types of cells to the site. These cells have specific jobs that are designed to remove whatever is causing the irritation and help the tissue that's been injured to start to heal. See Chapter Two for a discussion of the inflammation response and periodontal disease.

Interleukin A type of protein used in the immune system to stimulate the growth of cells that fight off disease.

Low birth weight A baby born weighing under 2,500 grams, or about five pounds eight ounces. Very low birth weight is under 1,500 grams or three pounds four ounces.

Macrovascular Pertaining to the body's major arteries and veins. These are the sites for arterial plaques and blood clots which can cause heart attack or stroke.

Microvascular Involving the smallest structures of the circulatory system, including venules, capillaries and arterioles. These connect with progressively smaller pathways, ultimately delivering nutrients to individual cells. In these sites, damage can be done to the eyes, kidneys, and lower extremities, areas that are particularly vulnerable to effects of diabetes.

Paresthesia Odd sensations of the skin ranging from numbness to burning. Caused by glycated hemoglobin cells that damage the microvascular system and prevent it from delivering adequate nutrients to nerves and other tissues in the skin.

Periodontal ligaments Connective tissues that do just that – they connect the cementum and the gum to the alveolar bone.

Periodontitis Put in its most simple terms, periodontitis is gum disease. The literal meaning of the word 'periodontal' is straightforward – 'peri' means 'around', and 'dont' means 'tooth'. So, periodontal refers to the parts of your mouth that surround your tooth. The word 'periodontitis' refers to the diseases that affect these parts of your mouth. These are generally bacterial infections that attack the gums and other oral components. See Chapter Two for types of periodontal diseases.

Phagocytes Cells that can engulf and kill other cells, such as the bacteria that are attacking your gums in periodontal disease. With your normal defenses lowered by diabetes, the bacteria can enter the bloodstream and trigger the body's inflammation response as well as attack major organs such as the heart and kidneys.

Porphyromonous gingivalis One of the most common pathogens in periodontal disease. If you have periodontal disease the risk of being infected with this pathogen is more than 11 times greater. This bacteria enters the bloodstream and travels throughout the body, and is believed to play a role in developing coronary artery disease that can lead to heart attack or stroke.

Preterm Delivery A baby born before the 37th week of pregnancy. Very preterm delivery is defined as birth before the 32nd week.

Prostaglandin A group of hormone-like substances that play a role in a number of body functions, including the control of inflammation, which may be caused by pathogenic periodontal bacteria.

Meet Dr. Martin

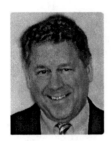

Dr. Martin is a senior diagnostician that teaches other doctors inside and outside the practice. He utilizes his extensive training and experience to treat even the most challenging dental situations. He has been delivering cosmetic, implant, and functional solutions to patients for over 30 years. His commitment to "doing it right" and ability to "handle just about anything" has won him the admiration of patients and other doctors. A big bonus is that Dr. Martin uses his expertise to prevent big problems from ever happening.

Training

- Graduate of Virginia Tech B.S. Biology 1975

- Graduate of Virginia Commonwealth University School of Dentistry 1979

Post Doctoral Training

- Misch Implant Institute

- Dawson Center for Advanced Dental Eduction

- L.D. Pankey Institute

- Summa Cum Laude Graduate of Cosmetic Dentistry

- Program at Case Western Reserve University

- Trained in many, many programs with the top dentists, both nationally and internationally

Teaching:

Dr. Martin has been an instructor at:

- Georgetown University School of Dentistry
- Medical College Of Virginia School Of Dentistry
- National Lecturer and Instructor for Other Dentists

Memberships:

- American Academy of Cosmetic Dentistry
- L.D. Pankey Foundation
- Academy of General Dentistry
- International Academy of Dentofacial Esthetics
- International Congress of Oral Implantologists
- Richmond Dental Society
- Virginia Dental Association

Recognitions and Awards:

Dr. Martin has a long history of achievement from his younger days in high school to college and now in his professional life.

As a Collegian, he was co-captain of the Virginia Tech football team, and received the Frank Loria award for scholarship and athletic achievement twice, was recognized by the ODK National Leadership Honorary Society, and the Who's Who in American College and Universities.

Now, as a dental professional, Dr. Martin has been awarded the designation of Fellow in the Academy of General Dentistry, Fellow in the American College of Oral Implantologists (Dental Implants), and Fellow in the International Academy of Dentofacial Esthetics (Cosmetic Dentistry). This is a very select dental-medical group that recognizes achievement in appearance enhancing care – making people look good. This special recognition is by nomination only and includes the top facial and appearance related health care therapists and researchers in the world.

Other Important Recognitions:

Master in the Academy of General Dentistry

This is a top-level honor coveted by general dentists available only to those who have first become a Fellow. It required several hundred hours of rigorous lecture and actual treatment of patients to meet its requirements.

Diplomate of the International Congress of Oral Implantologists

Dr. Martin is one of a very select group of Dentists awarded this international honor. He is one of the few dentists in the state to perform both the surgical and reconstructive phases on implant dentistry for over 20 years and with an impressive 90% plus success rate of treatment for that period.

Personal:

Born in Bristol, Virginia, Dr. Martin grew up in Bristol, Tennessee (literally across the street into Tennessee). He came to Richmond in 1975 after a successful education at Virginia Tech. He met his wife, Holly, on a blind date and was married on a steamy July night in 1977. They have 5 children – 4 girls and 1 boy (and yes, the boy was the last child!)

A Message From Dr. Martin

I have spent close to 10,000 hours in training in clinical dentistry, leadership, management and marketing. Thousands of those hours were spent outside my professional field.

Why outside dentistry? Because that is where the answers were to the problems that challenge you as a manager of a dental practice.

I have taught public speaking, sales, leadership, case presentation and communication. Over the past 20 years, I have consulted, coached and created programs for many different fields and professions: lawyers, accountants, painting contractors, a pharmaceutical equipment manufacturer, mortgage brokers, mortgage bankers, a pest control company, internet technology consultants, networking marketing experts, physical therapists, management consultants, marketing consultants, building contractors, and website developers.

I have helped them grow and manage their practices to discover their hidden, underutilized hard assets and underleveraged human capital. I have done the same for dental solo practitioners, group practices, implantologists and specialists in dentistry.

I have been a member of a mastermind coaching program outside of dentistry that has taught me the vast value of masterminding with a group of achievers. Members of that mastermind group encouraged me – no, challenged me – and demanded of me that I should create a mastermind group system for dentists.

I have added to it with leadership and coaching in a unique way to synergistically, geometrically expand the results far beyond anything else out there. That is why I'm so proud of this special leadership mastermind coaching program, which is unlike any other in dentistry anywhere. By design, only a limited number of dentists are allowed in the group so each gets individual attention.

Each of these previous endeavors was entered with a great deal of enthusiasm for the potential that lay ahead. I enjoyed them immensely and found them tremendously fulfilling, both personally and professionally.

Now, with this book I'm reaching out to the dental customer outside my practice area. It's crucial for you to understand the significant role good dental health plays in your over all health. It is an honor and a privilege to bring this book to you. I hope you find in it the tools to arm yourself with the knowledge you need to be a discerning dental customer. More importantly, I hope this book inspires you to become an active advocate for your own oral health so that periodontal disease never develops into a factor that damages your health

Most of all, I urge you to take the first step towards a healthy future and a long life by becoming your own dental advocate, by working with your dentist to get the care you need and enjoying your life to its fullest.

Contact Us:

Richmond Smile Center

11201 Huguenot Rd
Richmond, VA 23235
Office: 804-320-6800
Fax: 804.320.1014
Email: info@RichmondSmileCenter.com

www.RichmondSmileCenter.com
www.MartinSmiles.com

CPSIA information can be obtained at www.ICGtesting.com
Printed in the USA
BVOW03s1406271113

337535BV00015B/533/P